HOW TO CONDUCT SURVEYS

HOW TO CONDUCT SURVEYS

A Step-by-Step Guide

**Arlene Fink
and
Jacqueline Kosecoff**

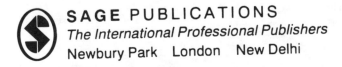
SAGE PUBLICATIONS
The International Professional Publishers
Newbury Park   London   New Delhi

For information address:

SAGE Publications, Inc.
2455 Teller Road
Newbury Park, California 91320

SAGE Publications Ltd.
6 Bonhill Street
London EC2A 4PU
United Kingdom

SAGE Publications India Pvt. Ltd.
M-32 Market
Greater Kailash I
New Delhi 110 048 India

Printed in the United States of America

Library of Congress Cataloging-in-Publication Data

Fink, Arlene.
   How to conduct surveys.

   Bibliography: p.
   Includes index.
   1. Social surveys. 2. Educational surveys.
I. Kosecoff, Jacqueline B. II. Title.
HN29.F53   1985   301'.0723   85-8170
ISBN 0-8039-2456-9

95 96 97 98 99 21 20 19 18 17 16 15

HOW TO CONDUCT SURVEYS

CONTENTS

Blest pair of Sirens, pledges of Heav'n's joy,
Sphere-born harmonious sisters, voice and verse

—John Milton

From the one with the voice to the
one with the verse,
and vice versa

PREFACE

The methods outlined in this book will help you organize a rigorous survey and evaluate the credibility of other ones. The methods are the basics or the "nitty-gritty" of surveys. We've taken some technical and not-so-technical material from many sources and hope nothing has been lost in the translation. Our purpose is to reach all those who need to conduct a survey, regardless of how skillful they are. We have aimed for simplicity, not for embellishment. We are confident that following the rules and principles of this book can result in sound surveys.

We are most indebted to a few people who helped us with this book.

Dr. David Kanouse's thoughtfulness can only have enhanced its quality; several of the book's omissions are probably due to our failure to pay full attention to Dr. Kanouse's remarks.

Dr. Wendy Everett Watson was a champ, a trouper, a true colleague. We took to heart her comments; we incorporated what we could into our book; she has no connection with any errors.

Thank you, David and Wendy. And thank you, too, to John, Robert, and the rest of the clan, whose strength is beyond "four-and-twenty men and five-and-thirty pipers."

We are grateful to the Literary Executor of the late Sir Ronald A. Fisher, F.R.S., to Dr. Frank Yates, F.R.S., and to Longman Group, Ltd. London, for permission to reprint Tables III, IV, and XXXIII from their book, *Statistical Tables for Biological, Agricultural and Medical Research* (6th edition, 1974).

—*Arlene Fink*
Jacqueline Kosecoff

1

CONDUCTING SURVEYS
Everyone Is Doing It

OVERVIEW

A survey is a method of collecting information from people about their ideas, feelings, plans, beliefs, and social, educational, and financial background. It usually takes the form of questionnaires and interviews. Used to help policymakers, program planners, evaluators, and researchers, surveys are most appropriate when information should come directly from people. Other information collection methods, such as observations, record reviews, and achievement and performance tests, may be more efficient for getting data from other sources.

Questionnaires and interviews share many of the same features. Both rely on directly asking people questions to get information, need instructions to be clear, must be concerned with who will be asked the questions (sampling), when and how often (design), and with the processing, analysis, and interpretation of data. Pilot testing helps get all survey methods in shape and can even help boost the response rate since a fair trial can help you keep the questions clear so that people do not get confused and give up.

To choose between questionnaires and interviews, select a method that is reliable, valid, and believable to the people who will be using the survey's results. Mailed, self-administered questionnaires are probably cheapest, followed by telephone interviews. Self-administered questionnaires can also guarantee anonymity, but if you need in-depth information and want to probe people's views, interviews are better.

Survey purposes and methods fall on a continuum. Some surveys can have far-reaching, generalizable effects, and their methods must be scientific. Others are conducted to meet very specific needs; their methods may not always achieve scientific rigor, but they must still be valid. This book aims to provide readers with the skills to conduct their own meaningful surveys and to evaluate others'.

WHAT IS A SURVEY?

A survey is a method of collecting information directly from people about their feelings, motivations, plans, beliefs, and personal, educational, and financial background. It usually takes the form of a questionnaire that someone fills out alone or with assistance, or it can be conducted as an interview in person or on the telephone.

There are at least three good reasons for conducting surveys:

Reason 1: *A policy needs to be set or a program must be planned.*

Example: Surveys to Meet Policy/Program Needs

- The YMC Corporation wants to determine which hours to be open each day. A survey of employees is made to find out which eight-hour shifts they are willing to work.

- The national office of the Health Voluntary Agency is considering providing day care for the children of its staff. How many have very young children? How many would use the agency's facility?

- Ten years ago, the language arts curriculum in the Bartley School District was changed. Since then, some people have argued that the curriculum has become out of date. What do the English teachers think? If revisions are needed, what should they look like?

Reason 2: *You want to evaluate the effectiveness of programs to change people's knowledge, attitudes, health, or welfare.*

Examples: Surveys in Evaluations of Programs

- The YMC Corporation has created two programs to educate people about the advantages and disadvantages of working at unusual hours. One program takes the form of individual counseling and a specially prepared self-monitored videotape. The second program is conducted in large groups. A survey is conducted six months after each program is completed to find out if the employees think they got the information they needed, whether they would recommend that others participate in a similar program, and how satisfied they are with their work schedule.

- The Health Voluntary Agency is trying two approaches to child care. One is primarily "child centered," and the children usually decide what they would like to do during the hours they are in the program. The other is basically academic and artistic. Children are taught to read, play musical instruments, and dance at set times during the day. Which

program is most satisfactory in that the parents, children, and staff are active participants and pleased with the curriculum's content?

- The Language Arts curriculum of the Bartley School District was changed. A survey is conducted to find out whether and how the change has affected parents' and students' opinions of the high school program.

Reason 3: *You are a researcher and a survey is used to assist you.*

Examples: Surveys for Research

- Because the YMC Corporation has so many educational programs, they want to research how adults learn best. Do they prefer self-learning or formal classes? Are reading materials appropriate or are films and videotapes better? As part of their research, and to make sure all the possibilities are covered, the corporation conducts a survey of a sample of employees to learn their preferences.

- The Health Voluntary Agency is considering joining with a local university in a study of preschool education. A survey is conducted of the participants in the agency's new day-care programs to find out about the participating parents' education and income. Data such as these are needed so that the researchers can test one of their major assumptions, namely, that parents with higher educations and incomes are more likely to choose the less academic of the two preschool programs.

- The Bartley School District is part of a federally funded national study of the teaching of the English language. The study's researchers hypothesize that what children are taught in the classroom depends more upon their teachers' educational backgrounds and reading preferences than upon the formal curriculum. A survey is conducted to find out teachers' educational backgrounds and reading habits so that data are available for testing the researchers' hypothesis.

WHEN IS A SURVEY BEST?

Many methods are available for obtaining information from people. A survey is only one. Consider the youth center that has as its major aim to provide a variety of services to the community. It offers medical, financial, legal, and educational assistance to residents of the city who are between 12 and 21 years of age regardless of economic or ethnic background. The program is particularly proud of its "holistic" approach, arguing that the center's effectiveness comes from making available many services in one location to all participants. Now that the center is 10 years old, a survey is to be conducted to find out just how successful it really is. Are participants and staff satisfied? What services do young people use? Is the center really a multiservice one? Are people better off in terms of their health and other needs because of their participation in the center? A mailed self-administered questionnaire survey is decided upon to help answer these and other questions. Here are some excerpts from the questionnaire:

**Examples: Excerpts from an Overly Ambitious
Questionnaire**

---

5. Is your blood pressure now normal?   11
   1. Yes
   2. No

7. Which of the following services have you   15-18
   used in the last year?

Services	Yes?	No?
(a) Medical	1	2
(b) Legal	1	2
(c) Financial	1	2
(d) Educational	1	2

10. Check how satisfied you are with each   20-28
   of the following services.

	1. Definitely satisfied	2. Satisfied	3. Neutral	4. Not satisfied	5. Def. Not satisfied
(a) Daily counseling session	1	2	3	4	5
(b) Legal aid facility	1	2	3	4	5
(c) Library	1	2	3	4	5

11. How much time in a five-minute period   29
   does the doctor spend listening to you
   (rather than, say, talking to you)?
     1. Less than a minute
     2. About one or two minutes
     3. More than two minutes

The questionnaire was shown to a reviewer, whose advice was to eliminate questions 5, 7, and 11, and keep only question 10. The reviewer stated that surveys are not best for certain types of information. Here's the reasoning:

Question 5 asks for a report of a person's blood pressure. Is it normal? In general, information of this kind can best be obtained from other sources, say, a medical record or directly from a doctor. Many people might have difficulty recalling their blood pressure with precision and also would be at a loss to define "normal" blood pressure.

Question 7 may be all right if you feel confident that the person's recall will be accurate. Otherwise, the records of the center (particularly if they are kept well) are probably a better source of information about what services are used.

Question 11 asks for how much time the doctor spends with the patient. Unless you are interested in a study of perceptions of time spent between doctor and patient, the best way to get this information is probably through observation.

Question 10 is appropriate. Only participants can tell you how satisfied they are. No other source will do as well.

Surveys are by no means the only source of information for policymakers, evaluators, or researchers, nor are they necessarily the most relevant. Some other sources of information are the following:

- observations or eyewitness accounts
- performance tests that require a person to perform a task (such as teaching a lesson to a class); observers assess the effectiveness
- written tests of ability or knowledge (these are usually used to tell if someone has learned or changed his or her attitude)
- record reviews that rely on existing documentation, such as audits of medical records in physicians' offices and hospitals and school attendance records

Surveys can be used to make policy or plan and evaluate programs and conduct research when the information you need should come directly from people. The data they provide are descriptions of attitudes, values, habits, and background characteristics such as age, education, and income.

Sometimes surveys are used together with other sources of information. This is particularly true for evaluations and research.

Example: Surveys Combined with Other Information Sources

- As part of its evaluation of child-care programs, the Health Voluntary Agency surveyed parents, children, and staff about their degree of participation and satisfaction. Also, the agency reviewed financial records to evaluate the costs of each program, and standardized tests were given to appraise how ready children were for school.

- The YMC Corporation is researching how adults learn. Achievement and performance tests are given at regular intervals. In addition, a survey provides supplemental data on how adults like to learn.

QUESTIONNAIRES AND INTERVIEWS: THE HEART OF THE MATTER

The most commonly used surveys are questionnaires and interviews. Questionnaires are sometimes designed to be self-explanatory, so that they can be filled out in privacy and without supervision ("self-administered"). Because of this, questionnaire forms are often mailed out to people rather than given to them in the surveyor's presence. Interviews are generally conducted in person or on the telephone.

Questionnaires and interview forms can look nearly identical because they share many important characteristics: They consist of (1) questions and (2) instructions, and they make sense only in the context of (3) sampling and design, (4) data processing and analysis, (5) pilot testing, (6) response rate, and (7) reporting results.

Questions

Information from questionnaires and interviews is obtained by asking questions (sometimes called "items"). The questions may have fixed or forced response choices:

Example: Fixed-Choice Item

What is the main advantage of using multiple-choice questions rather than essay questions in surveys?

*(1) can be scored quickly and objectively
(2) are best at measuring complex behaviors
(3) can have more than one right answer
(4) are the least threatening of the question types

Questions on questionnaires or interviews may be open-ended.

Example: Open-Ended Item

What is the main advantage of using multiple-choice questions rather than essay questions for surveys?

_____
_____
_____
_____

The selection, wording, and ordering of questions and answers requires careful thought and a reasonable command of language.

Instructions

For clarity, questionnaires and interviews should contain general directions. Are all respondents to answer all questions? Is there a time limit? Must all questions be answered? In a survey of viewers' television habits one section—for example, asking for the programs watched regularly—may be mandatory, while a second, calling for demographics or background information on age, educational level, and income, may be optional.

Survey Sample and Design

Questionnaires and interviews are data collection techniques that are used to obtain information from people. For which people, how often, and when? As soon as you raise such questions as these you must become concerned with the sample and design of the survey. The "sample" is the number of people in the survey. The "design" often refers to when the survey takes place (just once, or cross-sectional; over time, or longitudinal). Consider these three survey questions:

- Survey Question 1:

  What do college graduates know about physical fitness?

  Design: cross-sectional

  Sample: graduates from State College's class of 1984

  Method: mailed, self-administered questionnaire

- Survey Question 2:

  What do college graduates know about physical fitness?

  Sample: graduates from State College's classes of 1983, 1984, and 1985

  Design: longitudinal

  Method: mailed, self-administered questionnaire

- Survey Question 3:

  How has college graduates' knowledge of physical fitness changed over time?

  Sample: graduates from the class of 1984 surveyed in 1984, 1989, and 1994

  Design: longitudinal

  Method: mailed, self-administered questionnaire

Question 1 asks for a portrait of the class of 1984's knowledge of physical fitness, and a questionnaire is to be used. But must all graduates be included in the portrait? If only a sample is chosen, the survey will take less time and cost less. But will those in the sample think like everyone else? Fortunately, strategies exist for making sure that the sample is a microcosm of all graduates. If 40 percent of the 1984 graduates are male, and, of that, 10 percent are Hispanic, for example, it is possible to draw a sample that reflects these proportions and that is large enough to be meaningful, but not so large as to break the bank.

If the graduating class of 1984 contains only 100 people, and you can afford to survey all of them, then you do not have to worry about sampling; you will, however, be concerned with the fact that the survey is using a "cross-sectional" design in which people are surveyed just once, and that this is different from the longitudinal design in which people are surveyed more often. Question 2 calls for a longitudinal design because data are being collected from three graduating classes. To answer the questions about what graduates know about physical fitness, the three classes could be compared or combined.

The third question also calls for surveys over a three-year period and also uses a longitudinal design. In this case, however, the sample consists of students from just one graduating class and the survey is to describe how their knowledge or fitness changed.

All three surveys rely on mailed, self-administered questionnaires, but their designs and samples vary.

Data Processing and Analysis

Whether or not you plan to use computers, you must think ahead to how you plan to analyze the survey's data.

Will you compute percentages so that your results will look like this?

Of the total sample, 50 percent reported that they were Republican; 42 percent, Democrats; 5 percent, Socialists; 1 percent belonged to the Peace and Freedom Party; 3 percent had no affiliation; no one was affiliated with the American Independent Party.

Will you produce averages to appear this way?

The average age of the survey respondents is 56.4 years.

Will you compare groups?

A total of 60 percent of the men, but only 20 percent of the women, were Republicans.

No statistically significant differences could be found among respondents in their satisfaction with the present government.

Will you look for relationships such as this?

No connection could be found between how liberal or conservative people were and their educational backgrounds.

Will you look for changes over time?

> Since 1980, statistically significant differences
> could be found in the number of men participating
> in two or more hours of child care per day.

Pilot Testing

A pilot test is a tryout, and its purpose is to help produce a survey form that is usable and that will provide you with the information you need. All types of questionnaires and interviews must be pilot tested. Self-administered questionnaires are heavily dependent on the clarity of their language, and pilot testing quickly reveals whether people understand the directions you have provided and if they can answer the questions. A pilot test of a face-to-face interview will also tell you about interviewers. Can they follow the form easily? Are there sufficient spaces for recording responses? Pilot tests can also tell you how much time it takes to complete the survey.

Testing helps make the survey run smoothly. Whenever possible, you should try to duplicate the environment in which the survey is to take place. That might mean obtaining permission from people to be in the tryouts, but not in the survey, even though they are eligible for full participation.

Response Rate

The surveyor wants everyone who is chosen to respond to all questions. Pilot testing helps improve the response rate because it can eliminate several potential sources of difficulty such as poorly worded questions and no place to record answers. Further, if the entire set of survey procedures was carefully tested, then this, too, could help the response rate. For example, if a telephone interview is planned, then a check should probably be made on the correctness of the telephone numbers and the appropriateness of the times for calling. Do you have available a current source of information on people's telephone numbers? Are you willing to make telephone calls at the time the survey respondents are available? Other ways of ensuring good response rates exist. Among them are keeping surveys short and providing incentives (such as payment for participating).

How high should the response rate be? If you are conducting a large, complex survey, you will want to use statistical procedures to answer this question. If your survey is relatively simple (say, it is a poll of teachers in a school or nurses in three hospitals), then you have to decide how many people you would need for the results to be believable. If there are 20 people who are eligible for completing a mailed, self-administered questionnaire, and only 10 respond, you may feel different from the way you would feel if, at another time, 200 out of 400 responded. Both surveys would have yielded a 50 percent response rate, but reporting on the views of 10 out of 20 people may appear less convincing than telling about 200 out of 400. Except when done statistically, the desired response rate tends to be entirely subjective and the general rule is "higher is better."

Reporting Results

Survey results are daily reported on television and in the newspaper. In much of the public's mind, a survey is a poll, usually of some, but not all, people about an issue of immediate political, social, or economic concern. Survey results typically look like this:

Example: Survey Results

If the election were held today, would you vote for Candidate X?

	yes	no	don't know
men	62%	18%	20%
women	10%	85%	5%

Or like this:

Example: Survey Results

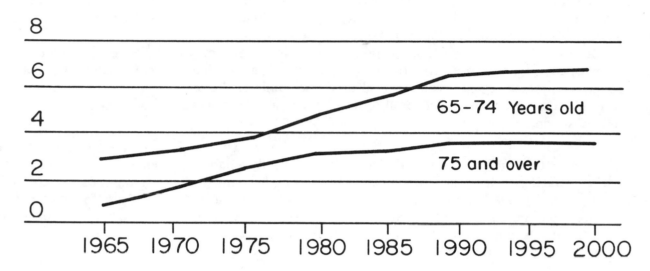

NUMBER OF APPLICANTS OVER 65 YEARS 1965-2000

Source: "A Survey of Applicants for Federal Programs," U.S.
Senate Committee on ABCD, 1984.

To get results such as these requires many steps, and all surveys follow them:

- deciding on the type of survey (mailed questionnaire, telephone, or face-to-face interview?)

- selecting the survey's content, writing questions, and trying out the form

- deciding who should participate (everyone? a sample of people?) and when (just once? each year for five years?)

- administering the survey (who should conduct the interview? By when must the questionnaire be returned?)

- analyzing and interpreting the results (Did enough people participate? What do the numbers or trends mean? Just how do people feel about Candidate X? Have opinions changed over time?)

- reporting the results orally or in writing in charts, tables, graphs

No credible survey can omit any single step although, depending on its purposes and resources, some steps will receive more emphasis in any given survey than in another.

QUESTIONNAIRES AND INTERVIEWS: THE FRIENDLY COMPETITION

Questionnaires and interviews are the most commonly used survey devices; they often look alike and can be used interchangeably. How do you choose between them?

Several fundamental differences do exist between questionnaires and interviews. With questionnaires, the survey is limited to written responses to preset questions. With interviews, it is possible to ask for explanations and to provide information on the respondent's reactions.

Here are some criteria for selecting among mailed, self-administered questionnaires and face-to-face and telephone interviews.

Reliability and Validity. These refer to the precision and accuracy of the information offered by the questionnaire or interview. Reliable and valid surveys are obtained by making sure the definitions you have used are grounded in fact or established theory or experience. Extensive pilot testing and analysis of the results will also ensure reliability and validity. Neither questionnaires nor interviews have greater reliability or validity to start with. Choose the method that is most precise and accurate for your specific purposes. For example, if you are worried that the people you are surveying cannot read well, an oral interview is likely to produce better results than a written questionnaire.

Usefulness or Credibility of Results. The results will be useful if they are reliable and valid and if the survey device is one that users accept as the correct one. Find out before you start which method is the one people want. Sometimes the people who will use the survey have strong preferences for or against interviews or questionnaires.

Cost. This refers to the financial burden of using the instrument. In general, questionnaires are less costly because they usually are mailed or handed out to people (say, in their office mailbox). For a given amount of money, you can usually cover the most people and the widest geographical area with mailed questionnaires. Telephone interviews and face-to-face interviews cover fewer people and less ground. But you must always make sure your mailing lists are up to date, since people move frequently in many parts of this country; telephone numbers change as people move, and, increasingly, many people are not listing their telephone numbers. Also, the response rate for questionnaires can be lower than for interviews, making the cost of either technique equal.

Anonymity. Questionnaires can preserve anonymity so that no one can trace the respondent. At best, interviews preserve confidentiality if the interviewer is unaware of the person's name (perhaps because he or she just has a telephone number or other identifying number).

Convenience. Questionnaires let people work at their own speed and when and where they want to. Interviews require more structure. Some say that the set order and time for completion mean that interviews produce more reliable information than questionnaires. Others have argued that, despite this advantage, interviews, by their very nature, contain a built-in bias because people react to the interviewer's style and not just to the questions.

Interviews may be extremely helpful to people who might ordinarily have difficulty with the self-administered questionnaire because interviewers can ask for clarification of terms.

Complexity of Information. Interviews have typically enabled respondents to provide more complex information than questionnaires because the interviewer can ask for explanations. (Why do you prefer. . . . ? What are your reasons for . . . ?)

A SURVEY CONTINUUM: FROM SPECIFIC TO GENERAL USE

Surveys are becoming a major means of collecting data to help answer questions about our health and social, economic, and political life. How extensive and scientific must a survey be?

All surveys, regardless of topic, scope, or method, share certain characteristics:

- They help set policy and formulate rules, provide data on the merits of services and programs, or offer new insights into thoughts and behavior.
- All surveys go directly to people for information.
- The reliability or the consistency and precision of information and validity, and the accuracy of information, are major concerns.
- Valid and reliable information is obtained by using the most rigorous methods available. This means having knowledge of survey design and sampling procedures and questionnaire construction.

- The results must be presented fairly and clearly.
- All surveys have at least two major contextual issues that guide how they are conducted. The first is adherence to ethical systems that respect the privacy of the individual and weigh it against the public's right to know. The second guide is the resources and constraints attendant on any survey project.

As a rule, surveyors with integrity attempt to shape their survey so that it looks like the model. In practice, however, some surveys are more equal to the model than others. This is especially true of relatively small surveys the immediate purpose of which is to provide useful data and which may not resemble the perfect model survey. It should never be true of those intended to provide information that could be used to affect the lives of many or make advances in knowledge.

Compare these two surveys:

Example: Survey with a Specific Use

The directors of the Neighborhood Halfway House want to provide services that are appropriate for residents. At present, many complaints have arisen over the lack of a physical fitness program and attention to other physical health needs. A survey will be conducted among the twenty current residents and three permanent and five part-time staff to see if services can be improved in these areas.

Example: Survey with General Use

The County Neighborhood Health Department is concerned with the merits of the ten halfway houses it supports. Together, the ten houses have over 1500 residents and 50 permanent and 150 part-time staff. A survey will be conducted to find out if services received by residents are appropriate and fairly and economically administered.

The justification for the first survey is one halfway house's concern with its own inner workings. The reason for the second is the supporting agency's concern over the merits of many houses. Survey 1, with its relatively limited impact, could probably be relatively informal so long as the directors are convinced of its usefulness. It may not even be necessary to preserve respondents' anonymity, for example. Survey 2, on the other hand, would have to be extremely careful about a sampling plan or response rate, the construction of the survey questionnaire, and how its data were analyzed and presented because many people would be affected. Usefulness is not the sole criterion for judging Survey 2; other criteria, mainly validity and generalizability, must be added.

Every time you do a survey, you make a judgment about where its purposes fall on a continuum that goes from having a specific use to a general one. All "generalizable" surveys must be conducted with rigor and automatically have the potential to be useful for many purposes.

The methods presented in this book are to help you produce the most rigorous surveys possible. Also, since surveys are used so frequently, we want you to be able to evaluate how credibly other surveys have been organized, implemented, and interpreted.

2

THE SURVEY FORM
Questions, Scales, and Appearance

OVERVIEW

To select the content of a survey, you have to define the attitude, belief, or idea being measured. For example, what is meant by fear? a liberal perspective? self-esteem? Also, ask, "What information do I need and must therefore make certain I will be collecting?" Choose content that people will give you because they remember the details and can and will give them to you.

Survey items may be closed- or open-ended. Closed-ended items with several choices are easier to score than are open-ended, short answer, essay questions. Open-ended questions give respondents an opportunity to state a position in their own words; unfortunately, these words may be difficult to interpret.

When writing closed-ended questions, use standard English; keep questions concrete and close to the respondents' experience; become aware of words, names, and views that might automatically bias your results; check your own biases; do not get too personal; and use a single thought in each question.

The responses to closed-ended questions can take the form of yes-no answers, checklists, and rating scales. Rating scales may be graphic, but often they ask respondents to make comparisons in the form of ranks (1 = top, 10 = bottom) or continuums (1 = definitely agree, 2 = agree; 3 = disagree; 4 = definitely disagree). The numerical values assigned to rating scales can be classified as nominal, ordinal, interval, or ratio. Each has characteristics that must be considered when you analyze the results of your survey.

Surveyors are most often interested in responses to individual items such as the number of people who will vote for Candidate X or how often women between 65 and 80 years of age visit a doctor in a three-month period. Sometimes they are concerned with a score on a group of items that collectively represent respondents' views, health status, or feelings. Making scores meaningful by proving that high scorers are truly different from low scorers requires knowledge of (additive) scaling methods. Three commonly used methods create differential (Thurstone), summated (Likert), and cumulative (Guttman) scales.

THE CONTENT IS THE MESSAGE

Once you have decided that a survey is the method you want to use to gather data, you must consider the content or topics it will include. This is a difficult task because any single survey can encompass hundreds of ideas (or more). Deciding on a survey's content means setting the survey's boundaries so that you can write the correct questions.

Suppose you were the evaluator of a youth center and that your main task was to find out whether the program's objectives had been achieved. Say that one of the objectives was to raise young people's self-esteem by providing them with education, jobs, financial help, and medical and mental health assistance. Suppose also that you decide to survey the young program participants to find out about their self-esteem. How would you determine what content to include?

To select the content of a survey you have to define your terms and clarify what you need and can get from asking people about their views.

DEFINE THE TERMS

Many human attitudes and feelings, such as self-esteem, are subject to a range of definitions. Does self-esteem mean feeling good about oneself, and if so, what does feeling good mean? The surveyor can answer questions of meaning by reviewing what is known and published about a concept such as self-esteem, or he or she can define it for himself or herself. The problem with your own definition is that others may not be convinced of its validity. When using a theoretical concept such as self-esteem, it is probably best to adopt a respected point of view, and even, if possible, an already existing and tested survey form.

Of course, for many surveys you will not be measuring theoretical ideas, but even so, you must define your terms. Suppose you were assessing a community's needs for health services. The terms "needs" and "health services" would certainly require definition since you could define them with respect to the type and nature of services that are required (ambulatory care clinics? hospitals? home visits?) and how convenient (time of day when doctors should be available) or how continuous they should be (must the same doctor always be available?)

SELECT YOUR INFORMATION NEEDS OR HYPOTHESES

Suppose two surveyors choose the same definition of self-esteem for their evaluation study of the youth center. Depending on the circumstances, Surveyor 1 might decide to focus on self-esteem in relation to feelings of general well-being, whereas Surveyor 2 may be concerned with feelings of self-esteem only as they manifest themselves in school or at work. Certainly surveyors 1 and 2, with their different orientations, will be asking several different questions. The results will yield different kinds of information. Surveyor 1, with a concern for general self-esteem, might not even cover work or school and would not be able to provide data on these topics. Surveyor 2, with his or her special interests in school and work, probably would not provide information on participant self-esteem with respect to personal relationships. The messages revealed by each survey would clearly be different.

Say you were interested in whether participants in the youth center had their general self-esteem enhanced after two years' participation in the program, and that you have defined your terms to conform to an accepted theory of adolescent personality. To make sure you get all the data you need, you must ask the question: What information do I want and must therefore make certain I will be collecting? Remember, if you do not ask for it, you cannot report it later on!

Here are some typical questions that the evaluator of the youth center could ask:

(1) Is there a relationship between general feelings of self-esteem and whether the participant is a boy or girl?
(2) Do participants' self-esteem differ depending on how long they have been in the program?

These two questions suggest that the survey must get data on three topics:

● general self-esteem
● sex of participant
● length of stay in the program

If any of these topics was omitted, the surveyor of the youth center could not answer the two evaluation questions. After all, in this case the survey is only being done for the evaluation.

MAKE SURE YOU CAN GET THE INFORMATION YOU NEED

In some cases people may be reluctant to reveal their views. The evaluator of the youth center might find, for example, that young people are sensitive to questions about their feelings. In other cases, potential survey respondents may simply be unable to answer. Suppose you wanted to ask participants who had been attending the youth center for about six months about their attitudes toward school just before entering the center's program. Many may have forgotten. This inability to answer is a major problem with accurately predicting voters' preferences in the national elections. It usually takes time for people to settle on a candidate, and frequently, people legitimately change their opinions several times during a campaign. That is why the national polls keep producing results that differ among themselves and from one point in time to another.

If you cannot get the information you need, you should find an alternative source of data, remove the topic from the survey, or wait until you can appropriately ask the question in a survey format.

DO NOT ASK FOR INFORMATION UNLESS YOU CAN ACT ON IT

In a survey of a community's needs for health services, it would be unfair to have people rate their preference for a 24-hour emergency room staffed continuously by physicians if the community were unable to support such a service. Remember that the content of a survey can affect respondent's views and expectations. Why raise hopes that you cannot or will not fulfill?

Once you have selected the content and set the survey's boundaries, your next task is to actually write the questions. Write more questions than you plan to use because several will probably be rejected as unsuitable. First drafts often have items for which everyone gives the same answer or no one gives any answer at all. Before deciding on the number of items, sequence of questions, and coding requirements, you must be sure that you cover the complete domain of content you have identified as important to the survey. You may want to keep a list that takes a form such as the following one used by the surveyor of participant satisfaction with the Youth Center. As you can see, this survey will not cover staff sensitivity, but will focus instead on consideration, accessibility, and availability of services.

Example: Plan for Survey of Satisfaction with the Youth Center

Topics	Number of Questions
(1) *Staff sensitivity*	
*counselor usually listens	O
*counselor is available when needed	O
*appointment staff courteous	O
.	
.	
.	
(2) Accessibility of services	
*hours are convenient	⊬⊬
*public transportation	⊬⊬ I
(3) Consideration of participant's needs	
*translation assistance	⊬⊬
*ease of getting appointments	⊬⊬ I
*waiting times	⊬⊬ I
.	
.	
.	
(10) Availability of needed services	
*medical	⊬⊬ ⊬⊬
*educational	⊬⊬ ⊬⊬ II

WRITING ITEMS

Open- and Closed-Ended Questions

Survey items may take the form of questions:

Example: Open-Ended Question

(1) How courteous are the people who make your appointments?

_____

_____

_____

Or they may be worded as statements:

Example: Closed-Ended Question

Circle your agreement or disagreement with the following:

(2) The people who make my appointments are courteous.
 (a) definitely agree
 (b) agree
 (c) disagree
 (d) definitely disagree

Sometimes survey items are open-ended, meaning that the respondents agree to answer the question or respond to the statement in their own words. Question 1 is open-ended. At other times, survey items are "closed" and force the respondent to choose from preselected alternatives as in Question 2.

The overwhelming majority of surveys rely on multiple-choice or closed-ended questions (also called "forced choice") because they have proven themselves to be the more efficient and ultimately more reliable. Their efficiency comes from being easy to use, score, and code (for analysis by computer). Also, their reliability is enhanced because of the uniform data they provide since everyone responds in terms of the same options (agree or disagree; frequently or infrequently; and so on).

Open-ended questions can offer insight into why people believe the things they do, but interpreting them can be extremely difficult unless they are accompanied by an elaborate coding system and people are trained to classify the data they get within the system.

Consider these two answers to a question from a survey of participants in an elementary school teaching program.

Example: Open-Ended Question for Elementary School Teaching Program

---

Question: What were the three most useful parts of the program?

_____

_____

_____

Answers: Respondent A
 Instructor's lectures
 The field experience
 Textbook

 Respondent B
 Instructor
 Teaching in the classroom
 The most useful part was the excellent atmosphere for learning provided by the program.

It is not easy to compare A's and B's responses. Respondent B lists the instructor as useful. Does this mean that the instructor is a useful resource in general, and how does this compare with Respondent A's view that the instructor's lectures were useful? In other words, are A and B giving the same answer? Respondent A says the textbook was useful. If only one text was used in the program, then A and B gave the same answer. But since the two recorded responses are different, some guessing or interpretation of what is meant is necessary.

Respondents A and B each mentioned something that the other did not: field experience and learning atmosphere. If these were equally important, then they could be analyzed individually. But suppose neither was particularly significant from the perspective of the survey's users. Would they then be assigned to a category labeled something like "miscellaneous"? Categories called miscellaneous usually are assigned all the difficult responses, and before you know it, miscellaneous can become the largest category of all.

Although it may be relatively easy for a respondent to answer an open-ended question, analysis and interpretation are quite complicated. The following closed-ended question could have been used to obtain the same information with the added result of making the responses easy to interpret.

Example: Closed-Ended Question for Elementary School Teaching Program

	Definitely not satisfied	Not satisfied	Satisfied	Definitely satisfied
(a) The textbook, *Teaching in the Classroom*	4	3	2	1
(b) The instructor's knowledge of subject matter	4	3	2	1
(c) The practicality of lecture topics	4	3	2	1
(d) The field experience	4	3	2	1
(e) Other, specify	4	3	2	1

ORGANIZING RESPONSES TO OPEN-ENDED SURVEY ITEMS: DO YOU GET ANY SATISFACTION?

A very common use of a survey is to find out whether people are satisfied with a new product, service, or program. Their opinions provide important insights into why new ideas or ways of doing things do or do not get used.

One open-ended set of questions that is particularly appropriate for getting at satisfaction requires collecting information about what people like best (LB) about the product or the service and what they like least (LL).

Here is how the LB/LL technique works:

Step 1

Ask respondents to list what is good and what is bad. Always set a limit on the number of responses: "List at least one thing, but no more than three things, you liked best about the conference." If participants cannot come up with three responses, they can leave blank spaces or write "none." If they give more than three you can keep or discard the extras, depending on the information you need.

Instead of asking about the conference as a whole, you may want to focus on some particular aspect: "List at least one thing, but no more than three things, you liked best about the workshops."

Step 2: Coding LB/LL Data

Once you have all the responses, the next step is to categorize and code them. To do this, you can create categories based on your review of the responses, or you can create categories based on past experience with similar programs.

Try to keep the categories as precise as possible—that is, more categories rather than fewer—because it is easier to combine them later if necessary than it is to break them up.

Suppose these were typical answers participants gave to the question on what they liked least about the conference:

- Some people did all the talking.
- The instructor didn't always listen.
- I couldn't say anything without being interrupted.
- Too much noise and confusion.
- Some participants were ignored.
- The instructor didn't take control.
- I didn't get a chance to say anything.
- Smith and Jones were the only ones who talked.
- The instructor didn't seem to care.
- I couldn't hear myself think.

You might categorize and code these answers as follows:

Example LB/LL: Response Categories

	Code
Instructor didn't listen (ignored participants; didn't seem to care)	1
Some people monopolized discussion (did all the talking; couldn't say anything; Smith and Jones were the only ones who talked)	2

Example LB/LL: Response Categories

Disorderly environment   3
    (too much noise; instructor didn't take
    control; couldn't hear myself think)

Now match your codes and the responses:

Example LB/LL: Participant Responses

	Code
Participant A	
Instructor didn't always listen	1
I couldn't hear myself think	3
I couldn't say anything without being interrupted	2
Participant B	
Instructor didn't always listen	1
The instructor didn't take control when things got noisy	3
The instructor ignored some students	3
Participant C	
I didn't get a chance to say anything	2

To make sure you assigned the codes correctly, you may want to establish their reliability. Are they clear enough so that at least two raters would assign the same code for a given response?

Step 3: LB/LL Data

When you are satisfied about reliability, the next step is to count the number of responses for each code.

Here's how to do this for ten participants:

Example LB/LL: Number of Responses for Each Code

	Codes			
Ten Participants	*1*	*2*	*3*	*Total*
A	1	1	1	3
B	1		2	3
C		2	1	3
D		1	2	3
E		3		3
F		2	1	3
G		2	1	3
H		2	1	3
I		3	2	5
J		1		1
	2	17	11	30

Look at the number of responses in each category. The ten participants listed a total of thirty things they liked least about the small group discussion. Seventeen out of thirty (more than 50 percent) were assigned to the same category, code 2, and the surveyor could justly argue that, based on the data, what the participants tended to like least about the workshops was that some people monopolized the discussions and others did not get a chance to say anything.

Next, count the *number of* participants whose answers were assigned to each code. For example, only participants A and B gave answers that were coded 1.

Example LB/LL: Participants' Response Pattern

Code	Number of participants listing a response assigned to this code	Which participants?
1	2	A,B
2	9	All but B
3	8	All but E and J

Look at the number of participants whose responses fit each category. Since eight or nine of the ten participants gave responses that fell into the same two categories (code 2 and 3), their opinions probably represent those of the entire group. It is safe to add that participants also disliked the disorderly atmosphere that prevailed during the workshops. They complained that the noise made it hard to think clearly, and the instructor did not take control.

When respondents agree with one another, there will only be a few types of answers, and these will be listed by many people. If respondents disagree, many different kinds of answers will turn up on their lists, and only a few people (fewer than 10 percent) will be associated with each type.

Interpreting LB/LL data gets more complex when you have many participants and responses to categorize. Suppose, for example, you asked 100 participants to indicate which aspects of a health education program they liked best.

First you must decide on your response categories and assign each one a code. Then try this:

(1) Put the codes in rank order. That is, if the largest number of participants chose responses that are assigned to code 3, list code 3 first.
(2) Calculate the percentage of students assigned to each code. If 40 out of 100 students made responses that were assigned a code of 3, then the calculation would be 40 percent.
(3) Count the number of responses assigned to each code.
(4) Calculate the percentage of responses assigned to each code. If 117 responses from a total of 400 were assigned to code 3, then 29.25 percent or *117/400* of responses were for code 3.
(5) Calculate the cumulative percentage of responses by adding the percentages together: 29.25 percent plus 20.25 percent = 49.50 percent.

Here is a table that summarizes these steps with some hypothetical data.

Example LB/LL: Summary of Responses

Response categories (with codes arranged in rank order)	Percentage of participants assigned to each code (100 participants)	Number of responses assigned to each code (400 responses)	Percentage of responses assigned to each code	Cumulative percentage of responses assigned to each code
3	40.0	117	29.25	29.25
4	34.0	81	20.25	49.50
7	32.0	78	19.50	69.00
8	20.0	35	8.75	77.75
10	17.0	30	7.50	85.25
1	15.0	29	7.25	92.50
6	10.0	14	3.50	96.00
2	5.0	10	2.50	98.50
9	3.0	5	1.25	99.75
5	1.0	1	0.25	100.00

You could then illustrate your findings graphically, as shown here:

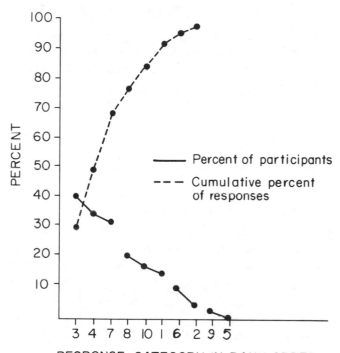

As you can see, the response categories are rank ordered along the X-axis according to the number of participants assigned to each code. The Y-axis represents percentages.

For each response category, you should look for two points on the X-axis: the percentage of participants and the cumulative percentage of responses. First, the cumulative percentages of responses are joined with a dashed line. Next, some of the points representing percentages of participants are joined with a solid line, grouping them as they seem to appear naturally on the graph.

The graph shows that responses coded as 3, 4, and 7 seem to cluster together. They are the categories to be emphasized because the highest percentages of participants were assigned to these codes, and they account for a total of 69 percent of all responses.

Items 8, 10, and 1 form a second intuitive cluster that represents 23.5 percent of all responses. Taken together, responses coded as 3, 4, 7, 8, 10, and 1 account for 92.5 percent of the total.

RULES FOR WRITING SURVEY ITEMS WITH FORCED CHOICES

Multiple choice, closed-ended survey questions consist of a stem, which presents a problem (typically in the form of a statement, a question, a brief case history, or situation) followed by several alternative choices or solutions. Here are rules for their construction.

(1) *Each Question Should Be Meaningful to Respondents.* In a survey of political views, the questions should be about the political process, parties, candidates, and so on. If you introduce other questions that have no readily obvious purpose, such as those about age or sex, you might want to explain why they are being asked: "We are asking some personal questions so that we can look for connections between people's backgrounds and their views. . . ."

(2) *Use Standard English.* Because you want an accurate answer to each survey item, you must use conventional grammar, spelling, and syntax. Avoid specialized words (unless you are testing people's knowledge of them) and abbreviations, and make sure that your items are not so lengthy that you are actually testing reading or vocabulary.

Example: Item-Writing Skills—Length, Clarity, Abbreviations, and Jargon

---

Length

Poor: The paucity of psychometric scales with high degrees of stability and construct validity is most bothersome to surveyors when measuring people's:
    (1) economic characteristics
    (2) feelings
    (3) knowledge
    (4) health

Better: The lack of reliable and valid methods causes surveyors the most problems when measuring people's:
    (1) economic characteristics
    (2) feelings
    (3) knowledge
    (4) health

Clarity

Poor: What remedy do you usually use for stomachaches?

Better: Which brand of medicine do you usually use for stomachaches?

Better: Do you usually use tablets or powder for stomachaches?

Abbreviations

Poor: Which political party is responsible for the diminishing size of the GNP?
    (1) Republican
    (2) Democrat

Better: Which political party is responsible for the diminishing size of the gross national product?
    (1) Republican
    (2) Democrat

Jargon

Poor: In your view, which dyad is most responsible for feelings of trust in early childhood?
    (1) mother and father
    (2) father and sibling
    (3) mother and sibling

Better: In your view, which family combination is most responsible for feelings of trust in early childhood?
    (1) mother and father
    (2) father and sibling
    (3) mother and sibling

---

(3) *Make Questions Concrete.* Questions should be close to the respondent's personal experience.

Example: Item Writing Skills—Concrete Questions

Less concrete: Did you enjoy the book?

More concrete: Have you recommended the book to anyone else?

More concrete: In the last year, have you ready any other book?

Asking respondents if they enjoy a book is more abstract than asking if they recommended it to others or read more books by the same author. The farther you remove a question from a respondent's direct experience, the closer you come to the problems associated with remembering.

Consider this:

Example: Item Writing Skills—Specificity of Questions

A survey of attitudes toward hiring women for managerial positions in five companies was conducted in a small city. Among the questions asked was, "Do you think women have as good a chance as men for managerial positions?" A friend of the surveyor pointed out that a better way of asking the question was, "At (fill in name of company), do women have as good a chance as men for managerial positions?"

Be careful not to err on the concrete side. If you ask people how many hours of television they watched each day for the past week, you should be sure that no reason exists for believing that the past week was unusual so that the data would not be representative of a "true" week's worth of TV viewing. Among the factors that might affect viewers' habits are television specials such as the Olympics, an event associated with the space program, and special movies.

(4) *Avoid Biased Words and Phrases.* Certain names, places, and views are emotionally charged.

When included in a survey, they unfairly influence people's responses. Words such as communist, president, George Washington, dope addict, and drunkard are examples.

Suppose you were surveying people who had just been through a diet program. Which words should you use: thin or slender; portly, heavy, or fat?

Remember this?

I am firm.

You are stubborn.

He is a pig-headed fool.

Look at these questions.

Would you vote for Roger Fields?

Would you vote for Dr. Roger Fields?

Would you vote for Roger Fields, a liberal?

Although Roger Fields appears to be the most neutral description of the candidate, it may be considered the least informative. Yet the introduction of Dr. or liberal may bias the responses.

(5) *Check Your Own Biases.* An additional source of bias is present when survey writers are unaware of their own position toward a topic. Look at this:

Example: Item Writing Skills—Hidden Biases

Poor: Do you think the United States and the Soviet Union will soon reach a greater degree of mutual understanding?

Poor: Do you think the United States and the Soviet Union will continue their present poor level of mutual understanding?

When you are asking questions that you suspect encourage strong views on either side, it is helpful to have them reviewed. Ask your reviewer if the wording is unbiased and acceptable to persons holding contrary opinions. For a survey of people's views on the relationship between the United States and the Soviet Union, you might ask:

Example: Item Writing Skills—Hidden Biases

Better: In your opinion, in the next four years, how is the relationship between the U.S. and the Soviet Union likely to change?
    (1) much improvement
    (2) some improvement
    (3) no real change
    (4) some worsening
    (5) much worsening
    (6) no opinion/impossible to predict

---

(6) *Do Not Get Too Personal.* Another source of bias may result from questions that may insult the respondent. Questions such as, "How much do you earn each year?" "Are you single or divorced?" "How do you feel about your teacher, counselor, or doctor?" are personal and may offend some people who might then refuse to give the true answers. When personal information is essential to the survey, you can ask questions in the least emotionally charged way if you provide categories of responses.

Example: Item Writing Skills—Very Personal Questions

Poor: What was your annual income last year?
    $ _____

Better: In which category does your income last year fit best?
    (1) below $10,000
    (2) between $10,000 and $20,000
    (3) between $20,001 and $40,000
    (4) between $40,001 and $75,000
    (5) over $75,001

Categories of responses are generally preferred for very sensitive questions because they do not specifically identify the respondent and appear less personal.

(7) *Each Question Should Have Just One Thought.* Do not use questions in which a respondent's truthful answer could be both yes and no at the same time or agree and disagree at the same time.

Example: Item Writing Skills—One Thought per Question

Poor: Should the United States cut its military or domestic spending?
    (1) yes
    (2) no
    (3) don't know

Better: Should the United States substantially reduce its military spending?
    (1) yes
    (2) no
    (3) don't know

or

Should the United States allocate more money to domestic programs?
    (1) yes
    (2) no
    (3) don't know

or

If the United States reduced its military spending, should it use the funds for domestic programs?
    (1) yes
    (2) no
    (3) don't know

TYPES OF RESPONSES FOR SURVEY ITEMS WITH FORCED CHOICES

Yes and No

The responses in a survey with forced-choice questions can take several forms.

Example: Yes and No Responses

Have you graduated from college?
    (1) yes
    (2) no

Does your car have front-wheel steering?
    (1) yes
    (2) no
    (3) don't know

Yes and no responses are simple to use and score. But a slight misinterpretation means that the answer will be exactly opposite from what the respondent really means. Also, in some cases, asking for absolutely negative or positive views may result in the participant's refusal to answer.

Checklist

A checklist provides respondents with a series of answers. They may choose just one or more answers depending on the instructions.

Example: Checklist Responses in Which Respondent Must Choose

(One Answer Only)

Which of the following medicines do you prefer most for treating a simple headache?

                                    (Circle One)

Aspirin 1
Tylenol 2
Anacin 3
Excedrin 4
Other, specify _____ 5
      _____

I don't take medicine for headaches 9

Example: Checklist Responses that Respondents Can Check

(Several Answers)

Check which of the following medicines you have taken during the past month.

	(1) Took this	(2) Did not take this
(a) Aspirin	_____	_____
(b) Codeine	_____	_____
(c) Penicillin	_____	_____
(d) Morphine	_____	_____
(e) Corticosteroids	_____	_____
(f) Cimetidine	_____	_____

Checklists help remind respondents of some things they might have forgotten. If you simply asked people to list their medications, chances are some would forget what they have taken. Also, checklists provide the spelling for difficult words. A problem with them is that the respondent might think a choice is familiar when it is not. Did they take penicilin or ampicillin? Was it this month or last? Also, it is somewhat difficult to format and interpret responses to checklists where multiple answers can be given. Suppose in the second example that a person checks aspirin and codeine, but fails to indicate whether or not the other medicines were taken. Can you assume that the others were not taken, or is it possible that they were, but the person did not bother to complete the item?

The Rating Scale

With rating scales, the respondent places the item being rated at some point along a continuum or in any one of an ordered series of categories; A numerical value is assigned to the point or category. There are four types of rating or measurement scales.

(1) *Nominal.* These are sometimes called categorical responses and refer to answers given by people about the groups to which they belong: sex, religious affiliation, school, or college last attended.

Example: Nominal Rating Scale

What is the newborn's sex?

                                      (Circle One)

Male 1
Female 2

(2) *Ordinal.* These responses require that respondents place answers in rank order. A person's economic status (high, medium, or low) would provide an ordinal measurement. A measure of whether an individual strongly agreed with a statement, agreed, disagreed, or strongly disagreed is considered an ordinal measure by some people and interval measure by others.

Example: Ordinal Rating Scale

What is the highest level of education that you achieved?

                                                    (Circle One)

Elementary school 1
Some high school 2
High school graduate 3
Some college 4
College graduate 5
Postgraduate 6

---

(3) *Interval.* With these measurement choices, distances between numbers have a real meaning. Annual income, for example, may be placed in intervals. The $10,000 difference between $20,000 and $30,000 a year means the same as the difference between $50,000 and $60,000 a year. However, having an income of $20,000 does not automatically mean that you are twice as rich as the person whose income is $10,000. Too many variables intervene, such as the number of people in the family, eligibility for assistance, savings, home ownership, and so on, so be careful and consider ratio measurements.

Example: Interval Rating Scale

How many millions of dollars would you be willing to spend on a three-bedroom, two-bathroom house on one-half acre with a pool in Beverly Hills estates?

(1) $1,000,000 to $1,500,000
(2) $1,500,001 to $2,000,000
(3) $2,000,001 to $2,500,000
(4) Money is no object

---

(4) *Ratio.* Height and weight are ratio measures. If you weigh 120 pounds and I weigh 240 pounds, I am twice as heavy as you. A ratio scale, like an interval scale, is one in which adjoining units on the scale are always equidistant from each other, no matter where they are on the scale. In addition, the ratio scale has a true zero. A ruler represents a ratio scale: the inch difference between seven inches and eight inches is the same as the difference between nine inches and ten inches, and zero means absence of length. With the ratio scale you can say that six inches is twice as long as three inches.

Surveys rarely have ratio measures. Usually only ordinal or interval scales are available.

Example: Ratio Scale

How many pounds did you weigh on your last check-up?

Weight in pounds: □ □ □

The distinctions between nominal, ordinal, interval, and ratio scales have more than academic interest. They determine the kinds of statistical treatments you can use: For example, the appropriate measure of "central tendency" for use with a nominal scale is the mode, whereas the median may be used with an ordinal scale and the mean with an interval or ratio scale (see Chapter 6).

Graphic Scales

For a survey of opinion on the city council's effectiveness in resolving certain issues, a graphic scale could resemble that shown in the following example.

Example: Graphic Rating Scale for Assessing a City Council's Effectiveness

Directions:

Make an X on the line that shows your opinion about the city council's effectiveness in resolving the following three issues:

	Very effective	Neutral	Very ineffective	
	1	3	5	7	9
(a) cleaning the environment					
	1	3	5	7	9
(b) new public transportation					
	1	3	5	7	9
(c) hiring teachers					

Graphic scales are a kind of rating scale in which the continuum of responses is visual. Because of this, you do not have to name all the points on the scale. In this example, only three points are identified: very effective, neutral, very ineffective.

Graphic scales are relatively easy to use. Be careful to put the description as close as possible to the points they represent. If you use the same scale twice for different parts of the questionnaire, be sure they have the same distances between points.

Item 10a is poor if used with 10b in the same survey

Example: Poor Formating of Graphic Scales

(10a)	Very effective			Very ineffective	
	1	3	5	7	9

(10b)	Very effective			Very ineffective	
	1	3	5	7	9

A major disadvantage of graphic scales is that they are sometimes hard to interpret. Look how these three respondents marked the same graphic scale:

Example: Interpreting Graphic Scales

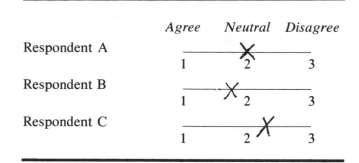

Respondent A has clearly selected a neutral rating. But what about respondents B and C? Both appear somewhat neutral, with B agreeing more than A and C, and C disagreeing more than either. You can decide to assign all ratings to the nearest point, in this case 2, or you can assume a true continuum, and assign Respondent B a score of 1.75 and Respondent C a score of 2.20. Since all graphic scales share this problem in interpretation, the surveyor will always have to decide on a strategy for making sense of the respondents' ratings.

Comparative Rating Scales

Comparative rating scales rely on relative judgments. The most common is the rank order, which is a type of ordinal scale.

Example: Rank Order Scale

Please rank the following five individuals according to their writing ability. The top ranked should be assigned the number 1 and the lowest ranked the number 5.

_____ Fay Gross
_____ Betty Bass
_____ Edward Romney
_____ Alexander Rulman
_____ Marvin Jackson

Another type of comparative scale enables you to contrast a single specific object in terms of a general situation.

Example: Comparative Rating Scale:

Please compare the Imperial Thai Restaurant to others in Los Angeles.

    (1) It is better than most.
    (2) It is about the same as most.
    (3) It is not as good as most.

To ensure that comparative rating scales provide accurate information, you have to be certain that the respondents are in a position to make comparisons. Do they have experience in judging writing skills? Are they fully acquainted with Thai restaurants in Los Angeles?

Category Scales

When raters use category scales, they select one of a limited number of categories that are previously ordered with respect to their position on some scale:

Example: Category Scales

---

    (1) frequently
    (2) sometimes
    (3) almost never

    (1) very favorable
    (2) favorable
    (3) neutral
    (4) unfavorable
    (5) very unfavorable

    (1) strongly approve
    (2) approve
    (3) undecided
    (4) disapprove
    (5) strongly disapprove

    (1) definitely agree
    (2) probably agree
    (3) neither agree nor disagree
    (4) probably don't agree
    (5) definitely don't agree

Are category scales ordinal or interval? Technically, they are ordinal; for many survey purposes, they are used as intervals. In any case, they are easy to use and interpret. How many categories should there be? Some people use as many as nine categories and others as few as three (two is yes or no). An even number of choices, say four, forces the respondent away from the middle ground "neutral" or "undecided." But, the needs of the survey and skills of the respondent must determine the number of categories. If very precise information is needed, the respondents are willing and able to give it, and you have the resources to collect it, use many categories; otherwise, use fewer.

Consider these two situations:

Example: Selecting the Number of Categories

---

(1) A four-minute telephone interview was conducted to find out how often families with working mothers ate dinner in restaurants. The question was asked: "In a typical month, how often does your family eat dinner in a restaurant?" The response choices were "two or more times a week," "once a week," or "less than once a week."

(2) Physicians were asked to rate the appropriateness of a comprehensive list of reasons for performing selected surgical procedures such as coronary artery bypass graft surgery and gallbladder removal. An appropriate reason was defined as one for which the benefits to the patients outweighed the risks. A scale of 1 to 9 was used: 1 = definitely inappropriate, while 9 = definitely appropriate.

In Situation 1, the four-minute interview dictated short responses. In Situation 2, physicians were asked to use their expertise to give fairly refined ratings.

ADDITIVE SCALES

Most surveys are designed so that each individual item counts. In a survey of people's attitudes toward living in a trailer park, you might ask twelve questions, each of which is designed in itself to be used to analyze attitudes and therefore is scored separately. Suppose you collected information like this:

- length of time living in this trailer park
- ever lived in one before
- satisfaction with trailer's accommodations
- satisfaction with park's accommodations
- satisfaction with quality of lifestyle
- amenities in trailer
- age of trailer
- age of car
- type of trailer
- type of car
- age of respondent
- annual income

With this information, you could report on each fact individually or you could look for relationships:

- between age of respondent and satisfaction with quality of lifestyle
- between sex and length of time living in the trailer park

Other surveys are different, however, in that the items do not count individually; they must be combined to get a score.
Consider this:

Example: A Survey with an Additive Scale

Doctors at University Medical Center observed that many of their very ill patients appeared to function quite well in society. Despite their disabilities, they had friends and went to the movies, shopping, and so on. Other patients with similar problems remained at home, isolated from friends and family. The doctors hypothesized that the difference between the two groups of patients was in their psychological functioning and access to the resources that make life a little easier for everyone. As part of testing their hypothesis, they plan to give the two groups the Functional Status Inventory developed jointly by the Herbert Medical School and California University. After five years of study and validation, researchers at the two universities have prepared a survey on functioning for use with chronically ill patients. High scores mean good functioning; low scores mean poor functioning.

The methods used to produce an additive scale require sophisticated survey construction skills because you have to prove conclusively that high scorers are in actuality different from low scorers with respect to each and every item. When you use a survey that produces a single score, check to see if evidence is given that it means something.

Defining Additive Scales

Surveyors use the term "scales" in at least two ways. The first refers to the way the responses are organized for an individual question or "item" and the second to a score that represents a person's views on many items. Try this:

Example: A Survey of Foreign Language Skills

Circle the category that best describes your ability to speak each of the following languages.

	Fluent	Somewhat fluent	Not fluent
(a) French	2	1	0
(b) German	2	1	0
(c) Italian	2	1	0
(d) Spanish	2	1	0
(e) Swedish	2	1	0

For each item—French, German, and so on—an interval rating scale is used to organize responses. At the same time, by adding all five items together, a scale of language ability can be derived. A respondent who is fluent in all languages would be at one end of the scale, while one who is not fluent in any would be at the other. Suppose you assigned two points for each language marked "fluent," one point each for those marked "somewhat fluent," and no points for "not fluent." A person fluent in all five languages could get a maximum score of 10 points, while someone who was fluent in none would be assigned the minimum score of zero. In this book, this type of scale is called "additive" (because individual responses to items are combined). Among the most commonly used additive scales are the differential, summated, and cumulative.

Differential Scales

Differential scales distinguish among people in terms of whether they agree or disagree with experts. To create a differential scale for an idea such as equality of opportunity, for example, means assembling many statements (for example, "qualified men and women should receive equal pay for equal work") and having experts rate each statement according to whether it was favorable to the idea. You next compute the experts' average or median ratings for each statement. Then you ask respondents to agree or disagree with each statement. Their score is based on just those items the respondent agrees with. To get it, you look at the experts' average score for each statement chosen by the respondent, add the experts' averages, and compute the arithmetic mean to get the respondent's score.

Typically, the directions to users of differential scales go something like this:

- Please check each statement with which you agree.
     or
- Please check the items that are closest to your position.

Scoring a differential scale might take this form:

Example: Scoring a Differential Scale

Student A was administered the Physical Fitness Inventory and asked to select the two or three items with which she most closely agreed. These are the two items she chose and the experts' scores.

	Median scores assigned by judges
(1) Physical fitness is an idea the time of which has come	3.2
(2) Regular exercise such as walking or bicycling is probably necessary for everyone	4.0

Student A's score was 3.6 (the average of 3.2 and 4.0), which was considered to be supportive of physical fitness. (The best possible score was 1.0 and the worst was 11.0.)

Are there disadvantages to differential scales? Perhaps the most obvious one is in the amount of work needed to construct them. Also, you must take into account the attitudes and values of the judges whose ratings are used to anchor the scale and interpret the responses. The judges may be quite different from the people who might use the scale.

Summated Scales

A summated scale aligns people according to how their responses to controversial or debatable statements add up. Suppose a self-esteem questionnaire has a series of items that use the same interval rating scale (agree, neutral, disagree):

Example: Creating a Summated Scale for a Self-Esteem Survey

Please rate your agreement with each of the following statements.

Statements	*Disagree*	*Neutral*	*Agree*
(a) At times I think I am no good at all.	____	____	____
(b) On the whole, I am satisfied with myself.	____	____	____
(c) I often feel very lonely.	____	____	____
(d) My social life is very complete.	____	____	____
(e) My friends admire my honesty.	____	____	____

How would you compute a summative scale score for this questionnaire? First, decide which items are favorable (in this case, b, d, and e) and which are not (a and c). Next, assign a numerical weight to each response category. You might do something like this:

- favorable = +1 point
- neutral = 0 points
- unfavorable = −1 point

A person's score would be the algebraic sum of his or her responses to the five items. The answers Person X gave are shown in the example below.

Person X disagreed with item a, which is fundamentally unfavorable, and got a score of +1. For item b, the person was neutral and so earned a score of 0. Item c produced agreement, but it was fundamentally unfavorable; person X got a score of −1. There was agreement with item d, resulting in a score of +1 and a neutral response to e, producing a score of 0. Person X's summated scale score was +1 out of a possible total of +5. (A perfect score of +5 would have come about if Person X answered: a = disagree; b = agree; c = disagree; d and e = agree.)

Summative scales are also called Likert scales.

Cumulative Scales

With cumulative scales, people respond to a series of items by indicating the extent of their agreement or disagreement. How are cumulative scales different from others? In cumulative scales, the items are arranged so that an individual who replies favorably to item 2 also, by necessity, gives a favorable answer to item 1; one who responds favorably to item 3 also does so to items 1 and 2. A person's score is computed by counting the number of items answered favorably and placing him or her on the continuum that goes from favorable to unfavorable that the items, taken together, represent.

Here's how such a scale might work:

Example: Cumulative Scale

Check which of the following jobs young women should be encouraged to pursue.

Jobs	Pursue? Yes	No
(a) Nurse	_____	_____
(b) Computer programmer	_____	_____
(c) President of the United States	_____	_____

Interpretation:

A person with a score of 3 would encourage young women to seek all three jobs; a person with a score of 2 would stop with computer programmer; a person with a score of 1 would only accept nurse from this list.

Example: Scoring a Summated Scale

Statements	Person X's Response Disagree	Neutral	Agree	Is item fundamentally favorable (+) / unfavorable (−)?	Item score
(a) At times I think I am no good at all.	✓	_____	_____	−	+1
(b) On the whole, I am satisfied with myself.	_____	✓	_____	+	0
(c) I often feel very lonely.	_____	_____	✓	−	−1
(d) My social life is very complete.	_____	_____	✓	+	+1
(e) My friends admire my honesty.	_____	✓	_____	+	0

Summated Score = +1

Cumulative scales are also called Guttman scales. In actual practice, it is always difficult to produce a set of items that constitutes a true Guttman scale, and you need statistical expertise to create one. If you plan to use a Guttman-type scale, check to see that it is technically sound. A good rule of thumb is that no more than 10 percent of the responses should violate the Guttman pattern in which a favorable answer to any given item means favorable answers to all the items that went before it.

Is Additive Scaling Just for the Experts?

The answer is probably yes. It is very difficult to define and measure general attitudes, feelings, and ideas because there are many conflicting theories of personality and development. Lack of agreement prohibits all but the most skillful from attempting to translate the theories into the survey instruments with scaled scores. And even with skill, the costs of scientifically validating additive scales would be beyond many budgets.

The good news is that most surveys do not need to be scaled because your concern will be with each item. Look at these:

- A survey of medical educators is conducted to find out what courses in geriatrics should be required of nursing students.
- Club members are surveyed to find out the goals they believe the organization should pursue.
- College graduates are surveyed to find out the annual salaries they earn from their first full-time jobs.

In none of these surveys would single scores combining all items into an additive scale make sense. Knowledge of scaling principles, however, is probably important. You should also pay careful attention to the scales of surveys you may want to adapt for your own purposes.

3

GETTING IT TOGETHER
Some Practical Concerns

OVERVIEW

How long should a survey be? Length depends on what you need to know and how many items are necessary so that the data will be credible, on the type of survey (since self-administered questionnaires may be shorter than face-to-face interviews), on the time you have available for the survey, on the time respondents can and will take, and on your resources.

The first question on a survey should be clearly connected to its purpose; objective questions come before subjective ones; move from the most familiar to the least and follow the natural sequence of time; keep questions independent to avoid bias; put relatively easy questions at the end (particularly of long surveys), but put "sensitive" questions in the middle; avoid many items that look alike; and place questions logically.

Self-administered questionnaires require much preparation and monitoring to get a reasonable response rate. Consider sending respondents a letter before the survey begins and also at the time of the survey; offer to send results; keep questionnaires short; and consider incentives to boost response rates. Interviewers should fit in with respondents and need systematic, intensive training.

You should pilot test your survey to see that it can be administered and that you can get the information you need. Your main goal is a reliable and valid survey. Reliability refers to the consistency of the information you get (people's answers do not keep changing), and validity refers to the accuracy of the information or its freedom from error. (You might consider a measuring tape reliable if it says yesterday and today that you are 2 feet 3 inches tall. This measurement could however, be invalid if you are actually 5 feet 4 inches tall.)

One way to ensure the reliability and validity of your survey is to base your survey on one that someone else has developed and tested. Check the results, and ask if the survey has proven its reliability. Also, if it has more than one form, ask if the forms are equivalent. Finally, you may want to check if the survey is homogeneous or internally consistent. Not all surveys are concerned with homogeneity. Many times your main interest is in each individual answer to questions on the survey. In some cases, however, you might be concerned with respondents' scores on several items combined. When you are, homogeneity counts.

When using someone else's survey, check the validity. Predictive validity is a measure of the survey's ability to forecast performance; concurrent validity means the survey and some other measure agree; content validity refers to the accuracy with which the questions represent the characteristics they are supposed to survey. Construct validity is experimentally obtained proof that a survey that is intended to measure a specific feeling, attitude, or belief truly measures it.

How do you establish the reliability and validity of your own survey? By pilot testing it or giving it a trial.

When pilot testing, anticipate the actual circumstances in which the survey will be conducted and make plans to handle them. Choose respondents similar to the ones who will eventually complete the survey, and enlist as many people as you can. For reliability, focus on the clarity of the questions and the general format of the survey.

Pilot testing also bolsters validity because it can help you see that all topics are included and that sufficient variety in the responses is available—if people truly differ, your survey will pick up those differences.

The use of surveys and concern for ethical issues are completely interwoven. Surveys are conducted because of the need to know; ethical considerations protect the individual's right to privacy or even anonymity. Large polling organizations have issued statements of ethical conduct that are worth reviewing.

The federal government has specified the legal dimensions of informed consent, privacy, and confidentiality. If you receive a grant from the federal government, you may have to obtain clearance, which means proving the necessity and value of your survey to the Office of Management and Budget.

Most public and private agencies that conduct surveys, research, evaluation, or perform educational services have policies on informed consent and confidentiality.

LENGTH

The length of a survey form depends upon what you need to know and how many questions are necessary so that the resulting answers will be credible. Length also depends on the type of survey you are conducting. Self-administered questionnaires and telephone interviews are generally limited to thirty minutes and contain the fewest items, while face-to-face interviews can continue for over an hour and can include many items. Another consideration is the respondents. How much time do they have available, and will they pay attention to the survey? Relatively young children, for example, may only stay put for a few minutes. You must also consider your resources. A ten-minute telephone or face-to-face interview will obviously cost less than an interview lasting twenty minutes. Here are two situations illustrating how the circumstances under which a survey is conducted influences its length.

Example: How a Survey's Circumstances Can Influence Its Length

---

Situation 1: The local library is concerned that it continue to meet the needs of a changing community. In recent years, many more of its patrons are over 65 years of age, and a substantial percentage speak English as a second language. Among the library's concerns are the adequacy and relevance of their exhibits, newspapers, magazines and other periodicals, programs featuring new books and writers, and special interest collections concerned with such issues as health. A bilingual volunteer will be devoting two mornings and one afternoon a week for eight weeks to a 45-minute face-to-face interview with users of the library. A fifty-item survey form has been designed for the purpose.

Situation 2: The neighborhood library is also concerned that its services be appropriate for a population that is getting older and many of whom prefer not to speak English. The city has decided that the neighborhood library is not the only one that is changing and has agreed to sponsor a survey of its library patrons' needs. To minimize the amount of time that librarians and patrons will have to spend on the survey, a ten-minute, six-item, self-administered questionnaire is prepared by the central library office. Four questions are asked about exhibits, periodicals, programs, and special interest collections and two about the respondent's educational background and income. To facilitate the survey's efficiency, questionnaires are left at the checkout desk, completed at the library, and left with the local branch librarian who then sends it to the central office for analysis.

PUTTING QUESTIONS IN ORDER

All surveys should be preceded by an introduction, and the first set of questions should be related to the topic described in it. Look at this introduction and first question for a telephone interview.

Example: An Introduction to a Telephone Survey and Its First Question

Hello. I am calling from California University. We are surveying people who live in student housing to find out whether it is a satisfactory place to live. Your name was selected at random from the housing registry, a directory of students who have voluntarily listed their telephone numbers. Our questionnaire will take no more than four minutes. You can interrupt me at any time. May I ask you the questions?

The first question asks you about your overall feelings toward your apartment. Do you consider it [read choices]:

(1) definitely satisfactory

(2) probably satisfactory

(3) probably not satisfactory

(4) definitely not satisfactory

(9) [DO NOT SAY] no opinion or don't know / wrong answer

The interviewer starts off by saying that questions will be asked about satisfaction with students' housing, and the first question calls for a rating of satisfaction. After the first question, the order in which the interviewer reads the questions will depend on several considerations.

People sometimes respond best when the first questions ask for objective facts. Once they become used to the survey and more certain of its purposes, they will usually provide the answers to relatively subjective questions. Suppose you wanted to know about the success of a summer city clean-up program, for example. You might first begin by asking participants how they first heard about the program and how long they had been in it (two questions of fact), and then, ask how well they liked their job.

Questions should proceed from the most familiar to the least. In a survey of needs for health services, items can first be asked about the respondent's own needs for services, then the community's, the state's, and so on.

Questions of recall should also be organized according to their natural sequence. Do not ask very general questions: "When did you first become interested in jogging?" or "Why did you choose jogging over other physical exercise?" Instead, prompt the respondent and ask: "When you were in high school, did you have any interest in jogging? in college?"

Sometimes the answer to one question will affect the content of another. When this happens the value of the questionnaire is seriously diminished. Look at this:

Example: Ordering Survey Questions

Which question should come first?

A. How much help does your advisor give you?

or

B. What improvements do you want in your education?

Answer: Question B should come before Question A. If it does not, then advisor-student relations might be emphasized unduly simply because they had been mentioned.

How about this: Which question should come first?

Example: Ordering Survey Questions

A. How satisfied are you with the president's economic policy?

or

B. What is the quality of the president's leadership?

Answer: Question B should precede A because a person who is dissatisfied with the president's economic policy (and perhaps nothing else) might rate the quality of the president's leadership lower than otherwise.

Place relatively easy-to-answer questions at the end. When questionnaires are long or difficult, respondents may get tired and answer the last questions carelessly or not answer them at all. You can place demographic questions (age, income, sex, and other background characteristics) at the end since these can be answered quickly.

Avoid many items that look alike. Twenty items, all of which ask the respondent to agree or disagree with statements, may lead to fatigue or boredom, and the respondent may give up. To minimize loss of interest, group questions and provide transitions that describe the format or topic:

Example: Providing Transitions

The next ten questions will ask you if you agree or disagree with different planks of the Democratic Party platform.

Questions that are relatively sensitive should be placed toward the end. Topics such as grooming habits, religious views, and positions on controversial subjects such as abortion and gun control must be placed far enough along so there is reason to believe the respondent is willing to pay attention, but not so far that he or she is too fatigued to answer properly.

Finally, questions should appear in logical order. Do not switch from one topic to another unless you provide a transitional statement to help the respondent make sense of the order.

Here is a checklist of points to consider in selecting the order for the questions in your survey:

(1) The first question should be clearly connected to the purpose of the survey as defined in the introduction.
(2) For any given topic, ask relatively objective questions before the subjective ones.
(3) Move from the most familiar to the least.
(4) Follow the natural sequence of time.
(5) See to it that all questions are independent.
(6) Relatively easy-to-answer questions should be asked at the end.

(7) Avoid many items that look alike.
(8) Sensitive questions should be placed well after the start of the survey, but also well before its conclusion.
(9) Questions should be in logical order.

QUESTIONNAIRE FORMAT: AESTHETICS AND OTHER CONCERNS

A questionnaire's appearance is vitally important. A self-administered questionnaire that is hard to read can confuse or irritate respondents. The result is a loss of data. A poorly designed interview form with inadequate space for recording answers will reduce the efficiency of even the most skilled interviewers.

Here are some do's and don'ts:

- *Do:* Put just one question on a line. Leave plenty of space for responses.
- *Don't:* Squeeze several questions together. Do not abbreviate questions.

Response Format

The general rule is to leave enough space to make the appropriate marks. Here are several response formats.

Example: Response Formats

A. ✓ 1. yes
    ___ 2. no
    ___ 3. don't know

B. ① yes
    2. no
    3. don't know

C.   *Code*
    yes   ①
    no   2
    don't know   3

D.   yes   no   don't know
        ①   2   3

If you use the format shown as A, be careful to provide enough space so that this doesn't happen:

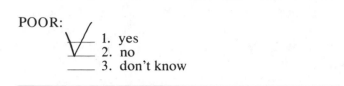

POOR:
_____ 1. yes
_____ 2. no
_____ 3. don't know

B or C is probably safer. D is not appropriate in this case, but would be for a situation such as the following where there are many statements being rated on the same scale:

	Yes	No	Don't know
(a) roses	1	2	3
(b) petunias	1	2	3
(c) gardenias	1	2	3

BRANCHING QUESTIONS

What happens when you are concerned with getting answers to questions that you know are only appropriate for part of your group? Suppose you were doing a survey of young people's participation in after-school activities. You know that one major activity might be sports and another might be music, but you also know that only some people participate in either.

If you want to ask about a topic that you know in advance will not be relevant to everyone in the survey, you might design a form such as the one in the following example.

Example: Branching Question

Do you participate in sports?
(1) yes
(2) no

If yes: Which sports do you perform?

	Yes	No
soccer	1	2
track and field	1	2
other, please name _____	1	2

OR

Do you participate in sports?
(1) yes   (complete section A)
(2) no   (go to section B)

With self-administered questionnaires, you must be extra careful in designing branching questions. Remember, respondents can skip important questions if they are confused about where to go next on the survey form. Interviewers must be trained to follow the branches or else they might be unable to administer the survey correctly.

ADMINISTRATION

Self-Administered Questionnaires

Self-administered questionnaires require much preparation and monitoring to get a reasonable response rate. These questionnaires are given directly to people for completion and very little assistance is available in case a respondent does not understand a question. A survey questionnaire asking about teachers' availability and needs for in-service training may be placed in their office mailbox, for example, with a week's return requested. Of course, teachers who have difficulty with the form might discuss the problem among themselves, but no guarantees exist that the solution will be just as correct or incorrect as if the individual acted alone. Mailed questionnaires isolate the respondents the most, since no one is usually available to clear up confusion.

Advance preparation, in the form of careful editing and tryouts, will unquestionably help produce a clear, readable self-administered questionnaire. To further ensure that you get what you need, you should review the returns. Are you getting the response rate you expected? Are all questions being answered? Here is a checklist for using self-administered questionnaires that can help you get what you need.

Checklist for Using Self-Administered Questionnaires

(1) Send respondents a preletter telling them the purpose of your survey questionnaire. This should warn people that the survey is coming, explain why the respondents should answer the questions, and tell them about who is being surveyed.

(2) Prepare a short, formal letter to accompany the questionnaire form. If you have already sent a preletter, this one should be very concise. It should again describe the survey and questionnaire aims and participants.

(3) Offer to send respondents a summary of the findings so they can see just how the data are used. (If you promise this, budget for it.)

(4) If you ask questions that may be construed as personal—such as sex, age, or income—explain why they are necessary.

(5) Keep the questionnaire procedures simple. Provide stamped self-addressed envelopes. Keep page folding to a minimum so respondents do not feel they are involved in complicated physical activities.

(6) Keep questionnaires as short as you can. Ask only the questions you are sure you need and do not crowd them together. Give respondents enough room to write and be sure each question is set apart from the next.

(7) Consider incentives. This may encourage people to respond. These may range from money and stamps to pens or food.

(8) Be prepared to follow up or send reminders. These should be brief and to the point. It often helps to send another copy of the questionnaire. Do not forget to budget money and time for these additional mailings.

Interviews

Finding Interviewers. Interviewers should fit in as well as possible with respondents. They should avoid flamboyant clothes, haircuts, and so on. Sometimes it is a good idea to select interviewers who are similar to respondents. If you want to find out why adolescent girls smoke, for example, you might hire young women to do the questioning.

It is also important that the interviewers be able to speak clearly and understandably. Unusual speech patterns or accents may provoke unnecessarily favorable or unfavorable reactions. The interviewer's way of talking is of course an extremely important consideration in the telephone interview. You should be keenly aware of the possibility that the interviewer's attitude toward the survey and respondent will influence the results. If the interviewer does not expect much and sends this message, the response rate will probably suffer. To make sure you are getting the most accurate data possible, you should monitor the interviewers.

Training Interviewers. The key to a good telephone or face-to-face interview is training, which should ensure that all interviewers know what is expected of them and that they ask all the questions in the same way, within the same amount of time.

Whether you are training two interviewers or twenty, it is important to find a time to meet together. The advantage of meetings is that everyone can develop a standard vocabulary and share problems. If the trainees have to travel to reach you, you may have to think about paying for gasoline or other means of private or public transportation.

Once at the training site, trainees must have enough space to sit and write or perform any other activities you will require of them. If you want them to interview one another as practice for their real task, be sure the room is large enough so that two or more groups can speak without disturbing the others. You may even need several rooms.

If training takes more than an hour and a half, you should provide some form of refreshment. If you cannot afford to do that, at least give trainees time to obtain their own.

Trainees should be taken step by step through their tasks and given an opportunity to ask questions. It is also essential to tell them some of the reasons for their tasks so they can anticipate problems and be prepared to solve them. The most efficient way to make sure the trainees have all the information they need to perform their job is to prepare a manual. Here you can explain what they are to do and when, where, why, and how they are to do it. A three-ring binder makes it easy to add pages, if necessary.

Conducting Interviews. Here are some tips on conducting interviews that should be emphasized in your training sessions:

(1) Make a brief introductory statement that will describe who is conducting the interview ("Mary Doe for Armstrong Memorial Medical Center"), tell why the interview is being conducted ("to find out how satisfied you are with our hospitality program"), explain why the respondent is being called ("we're asking a random sample of people who were discharged from the hospital in the last two months"), and indicate whether or not answers will be kept confidential ("your name will not be used without your written permission").

(2) Try to impress the person being interviewed with the importance of the interview and of the answers. People are more likely to cooperate if they appreciate the importance of the subject matter. Do not try to deal with every complaint or criticism, but suggest that all answers will receive equal attention.

(3) Flexibility is needed. Although it is important to stay on schedule and ask all the questions, a few people may have trouble hearing and understanding some of the questions. If that happens, slow down and repeat the question.

(4) Interview people alone. The presence of another person may be distracting and alter results.

(5) Ask questions as they appear in the interview schedule. It is important to ask everyone the same questions in the same way or the results will not be comparable.

(6) Interviewers should follow all instructions given at the training session and described on the interview form. Sometimes instructions involve a sequence of questions such as, "Ask Question 10 only if the answer to Question 9 is no," or "Ask Question 11 only if the answer to Question 9 is yes."

Monitoring Interviews. To make sure you are getting the most accurate data possible, you should monitor the interviewers. This might mean something as informal as having the interviewer call you once a week, or something as formal as having them submit to you a standardized checklist of activities they perform each day. If possible, you may actually want to go with an interviewer (if it is a face-to-face interview) or spend time with telephone interviewers to make sure that what they are doing is appropriate for the survey's purposes. To prevent problems, you might want to take some or all of the following steps:

- Establish a hot line—someone available to answer any questions that might occur immediately, even at the time of an interview.

- Provide written scripts. If interviewers are to introduce themselves or the survey, give them a script or set of topics to cover.

- Make sure you give out extra copies of all supplementary materials. If data collectors are to mail completed interviews back to you, for example, make sure to give them extra forms and envelopes.

- Provide an easy-to-read handout describing the survey.

- Provide a schedule and calendar so that interviewers can keep track of their progress.

- Consider providing the interviewer with visual aids. Visual aids may be extremely important when interviewing people whose ability to speak the language may not be as expert as is necessary to understand the survey. Visual aids are also very useful in clarifying ideas and making sure that everybody is reacting to similar stimuli. For example, suppose you wanted to find out whether or not people perceived that the economy was improving. To ensure that everybody had access to the same set of data on the economy, you might show graphs and tables describing the economy taken from the local newspaper for the last one or two years. Another use of a visual aid might be in a survey of people's ideal expectations for a planned community. You might show several different plans and ask people to describe their reactions to each. The preparation of audiovisual aids for use in an interview is relatively expensive and requires that interviewers be specially trained in using them.

- Consider the possibility that some people may need to be retrained and make plans to do so.

THE SURVEY IS PUT ON TRIAL

Once your survey has been assembled, you must try it out to see that it can be administered and that you can get accurate data. That means testing the logistics of the survey (the ease with which the interviewers can record responses) as well as the survey form itself. The purpose of the trial (sometimes called a pretest or pilot test) is to answer these questions:

- Will the survey provide the needed information? Are certain words or questions redundant or misleading?
- Are the questions appropriate for the people who will be surveyed?
- Will information collectors be able to use the survey forms properly? Can they administer, collect, and report information using any written directions or special coding forms?
- Are the procedures standardized? Can everyone collect information in the same way?
- How consistent is the information obtained by the survey?
- How accurate is the information obtained from the survey?

Reliability and Validity:
The Quality of Your Survey

A ruler is considered to be a reliable instrument if it yields the same results every time it is used to measure the same object, assuming the object itself has not changed. A yardstick showing that you are 6 feet 1 inch tall today and six months from now is reliable.

People will change, of course. You may be more tired, angry, and tense today than you were yesterday. People also change because of their experiences or because they learned something new, but meaningful changes are not subject to random fluctuations. A reliable survey will provide a consistent measure of important characteristics despite background fluctuations.

A ruler is considered to be a valid instrument if it provides an accurate measure (free from error) of a person's height. But even if the ruler says you are 6 feet 1 inch tall today and six months from now (meaning it is reliable), it may be incorrect. This would occur if the ruler were not calibrated accurately, and you are really 5 feet 6 inches tall.

If you develop a survey that consists of nothing more than asking a hospital administrator how many beds are in a given ward, and you get the same answer on at least two occasions, you would have an instrument that is stable and reliable. But if you claim that the same survey measures the quality of medical care, you have a reliable survey of questionable validity. A valid survey is always a reliable one, but a reliable one is not always valid.

Ensuring Quality:
Selecting Ready-to-Use Surveys

One way to make sure that you have a reliable and valid survey is to use one that someone else has prepared and demonstrated to be reliable and valid through careful testing. This is particularly important to remember if you want to survey attitudes, feelings, and beliefs. These factors, derived from the psychological or affective side of human development, have proven to be somewhat elusive and difficult to measure. To produce a truly satisfactory survey of human emotions thus requires a large-scale and truly scientific experimental study.

Some surveys are available for use, however, (possibly at a cost to the surveyor), and should always be considered. To find them you can:

(1) Contact the major publishers of psychological tests, the names of which can be obtained from local schools, a university's psychology department, or the library.
(2) Review the research literature.

In reviewing a published survey (also, in assessing the quality of a homemade form) you should ask the following questions about three types of reliability: stability, equivalence, and homogeneity.

First, does the survey have stability? One way to estimate reliability is to see if someone taking the survey answers about the same on more than one occasion. Stability is usually computed by administering a survey to the same group on two different occasions and then correlating the scores from one time to the next. This type of reliability is also known as test/retest reliability. A survey is considered reliable if the correlation between results is high; that is, people who have good (or poor) attitudes on the first occasion also have good (or poor) attitudes on the second occasion. How high should the correlation be? Not much agreement exists about what is acceptable, but the higher, the better. Look for correlations of at least .70.

Second, are alternative forms equivalent? If two different forms of a survey are supposed to appraise the same attitude, you should to make sure that people will score the same regardless of which one they take. If you want to use Form A of the survey as a premeasure, for example, and Form B as a postmeasure, check the equivalence of the two forms to make sure one is not different from the other.

Equivalence reliability can be computed by giving two or more forms of the same survey to the same group of people on the same day, or by giving different forms of the survey to two or more groups that have been randomly selected. You determine equivalence by comparing the mean score and standard deviations of each form of the survey and by correlating the scores on each form with the scores on the other. If the various forms have almost the same means and standard deviations and they are highly correlated, then they have high equivalence reliability. Equivalence reliability coefficients should be high; look for those that are as close to perfect as possible.

Does the survey have homogeneity? Is it internally consistent? Another measure of reliability is how harmoniously the questions on a survey measure the characteristics, attitudes, or qualities that they are supposed to measure. To test for harmony or, in technical terms, homogeneity, divide the survey into two equal parts and correlate the scores on one half with the scores on the other half. This procedure is called split-half reliability, and it estimates whether both halves of the survey measure the same characteristics. Another way to estimate a survey's homogeneity is to use the Kuder-Richardson Formula-20, also called coeffi-

cient alpha. This formula is really the average score obtained from computing all possible split-half reliabilities. If you are interested in homogeneity, look for high correlations.

Many surveyors are not at all concerned with homogeneity because they are not going to be using several items to measure one attitude or characteristic. Instead, they are interested in the responses to each item. Decide if your survey needs to consider homogeneity.

Example: Homogeneity or Internal Consistency Counts

A ten-item interview is conducted to find out patients' satisfaction with medical care in hospitals. High scores mean much satisfaction; low scores mean little satisfaction. To what extent do the ten items each measure the same dimension of satisfaction with hospital care?

Example: Homogeneity or Internal Consistency Does Not Count

A ten-item interview is conducted with patients as part of a study to find out how hospitals can improve. Eight items ask about potential changes in different services such as the type of food that might be served; the availability of doctors, nurses, or other health professionals, and so on. Two items ask patients for their age. Since this survey is concerned with views on improving eight very different services and with providing data on the age and education of respondents, each item is independent of the others.

Here are some questions to ask about a published survey's validity:

• Does the survey have predictive validity? You can validate a survey by proving that it predicts an individual's ability to perform a given task or behave in a certain way. For example, a medical school entrance examination has predictive validity if it accurately forecasts performance in medical school. One way of establishing predictive validity is to administer the survey to all students who want to enter medical school and compare these scores with their performance in school. If the two sets of scores show a high positive or negative correlation, the survey or instrument has predictive validity.

• Does the survey have concurrent validity? You can validate a survey by comparing it against a known and accepted measure. To establish the concurrent validity of a new survey of attitudes toward mathematics, you could administer the new survey and an already established, validated survey to the same group and compare the scores from both instruments. You could also administer just the new survey to the respondents and compare their scores on it to experts' judgment of the respondents' attitudes. A high correlation between the new survey and the criterion measure (the established survey or expert judgment) means concurrent validity. Remember, a concurrent validity study is only valuable if the criterion measure is convincing.

• Does the survey have content validity? A survey can be validated by proving that its items or questions accurately represent the characteristics or attitudes that they are intended to measure. A survey of political knowledge has content validity, for example, if it contains a reasonable sample of facts, words, ideas, and theories commonly used when discussing or reading about the political process. Content validity is usually established by asking experts whether the items are representative samples of the attitudes and traits you want to survey.

• Does the survey have construct validity? Surveys can be validated by demonstrating that they measure a psychological construct such as hostility or satisfaction. Construct validity is established experimentally by trying the survey on people whom the experts say do and do not exhibit the behavior associated with the construct. If the people whom the experts judge to have high degrees of hostility or satisfaction also obtain high scores on surveys designed to measure hostility or satisfaction, then the surveys are considered to have construct validity.

GUIDELINES FOR PILOT TESTING

Here are some basic rules for a fair trial of a survey.

(1) Try to anticipate the actual circumstances in which the survey will be conducted and make plans to handle them. For interviews, this means reproducing the training manual and all forms; for mailed questionnaires, you have to produce any covering letters, return envelopes, and so on. Needless to say, this requires planning and time and can be costly.

(2) You can start by trying out selected portions of the survey in a very informal fashion. Just the directions on a self-administered questionnaire might be tested first, for example, or the wording of several questions in an interview might be tested. You may also want to try out the survey process initially by using a different method from the one you eventually intend to use. So, if you are planning to hand out questionnaires to conference participants, the trial may involve an interview so that any problems with the questions on the form can be discussed. In the end, you should give the survey logistics and form a fair pretrial.

(3) Choose respondents similar to the ones who will eventually complete the survey. They should be approximately the same age, with a similar education, and so on.

(4) Enlist as many people in the trial as seems reasonable without wasting your resources. Probably fewer people will be needed to test a five-item questionnaire than a twenty-item one. Also, if you see that the survey needs little improvement, stop.

(5) For reliability, focus on the clarity of the questions and the general format of the survey. Here is what you look for:

- failure to answer questions
- giving several answers to the same question
- writing comments in the margin

Any one of these is a signal that the questionnaire may be unreliable and needs revision. Are the choices in forced-choice questions mutually exclusive? Have you provided all possible alternatives? Is the questionnaire or interview language clear and unbiased? Do the directions and transitions make sense? Have you chosen the proper order for the questions? Is the questionnaire too long or hard to read? Does the interview take too long? (For instance, you planned for a ten-minute interview, but your pilot version takes twenty.)

(6) To help bolster validity, you should make sure that all relevant topics have been included in the survey (given your resources). For a survey of political attitudes, have you included all political parties? Controversial issues? What else must be included for your survey to have content validity? If you are not certain, check with other people, including the trial-run respondents. Does the survey have room for the expression of all views? Suppose you were surveying people to find out how religious they were. If you had proof in advance that all were very religious, you would not need a survey. Unless you can show that at least in theory you can distinguish the religious from the nonreligious, no one would believe the results. How do you fix this? In the trials, choose people you know are religious and those you know are not and give them the survey. Do their responses differ?

(7) Test your ability to get a range of responses. If people truly differ in their views or feelings, will the survey capture those differences? Suppose your survey was of a suburban neighborhood's attitude toward a proposed new high-rise building development. You should administer the survey to people who are both for and against the building. This will help reveal your own biases in how questions are worded, and, for closed-ended questions, might help you identify choices that people who feel strongly one way perceive as missing, but that you might not have thought of.

Consider this:

In a pilot of a survey of children's attitudes toward health, respondents were asked how often they washed their hands after eating. All six children between 8 and 10 years of age answered "always" after being given the choices "always," "never," and "I don't know." The choices were changed to "almost always," "usually," and "almost never." With the new categories, the same six children changed their answers to two "almost always" and four "usually."

(8) If you must test your survey more than once, you probably can use the same people.

ETHICS, PRIVACY, AND CONFIDENTIALITY

The use of surveys and concern for ethical issues are completely interwoven. Surveys are conducted because of the need to know; ethical considerations protect the individual's right to privacy or even anonymity.

The National Council on Public Polls and the American Association of Public Opinion Research have rules for disclosure and codes that are important statements of ethical conduct. These are certainly worthy of review.

If your survey is for a public or private agency that is receiving federal funds, you should know that the federal government has specified the legal dimensions of informed consent, privacy, and confidentiality. These dimensions include:

- a fair explanation of the procedures to be followed and their purposes
- a description of any risks and benefits
- an offer to answer any inquiries
- an instruction that the person is free to withdraw consent and to discontinue participation without prejudice

Confidentiality is protected by the "Protection of Human Subjects" guidelines of the Code of Federal Regulations. Confidentiality refers to the safeguarding of any information about one person that is known by another. A surveyor who has names and addresses of people, even in coded form, must not use this information to reveal identities. In many surveys, confidentiality is a real concern because complete anonymity is virtually impossible. A code number or even sometimes just a zipcode can help lead to the survey respondent's identity.

If your agency receives a grant from the federal government, and you want to survey ten or more people in a ten-month period by means of identical questions, you probably have to obtain clearance from the Office of Management and Budget. Getting clearance means describing the data you will collect and justifying the need to collect it. You have to prove the following:

- You will collect the necessary information in a manner that puts the least possible burden on your expected respondents.
- The information you will collect does not duplicate data already accessible from the government agency supporting your grant.
- The information you will collect will be useful.

Clearance from the Office of Management can take sixty days (or in difficult cases, up to ninety days) and is granted for no longer than three years.

If you work for a private agency, organization, or business, you should check the rules of informed consent and confidentiality. Is there a committee whose approval you must get? If you are a student, check to see whether you can ask the questions you are planning. Also, you may be part of a larger project that has already received clearance for its activities as long as it conforms to certain standards. Almost all groups that sponsor research and evaluation activities, of which your survey may be a part, will have devised some controls.

4

SAMPLING

OVERVIEW

Should you survey everyone or just a sample? This depends on how quickly data are needed, what type of survey you are conducting, your resources, the need for credibility, and your familiarity with survey sampling methods.

Two basic methods of sampling are probability and nonprobability sampling. A probability sample is one in which each person in the population has an equal chance of being selected. The resulting sample is said to be representative.

In simple random sampling, you select people at random (using a table or random numbers, for example). It is fairly simple, but if your sample has certain subgroups that might influence the results, you have to use stratified random sampling. Cluster sampling is like random sampling except that groups, such as a classroom or school, are selected at random rather than individuals. You use it when sampling individuals is unethical or administratively difficult. Unfortunately, cluster sampling produces a small number of units to study. If, for example, you have 150 people in your sample, but they are in five classrooms of thirty children each, you only have a sample of five the results of which you can analyze.

Systematic sampling lets you choose every second, tenth, or nth number from a list, and the number can be randomly chosen. If the list has a pattern (say, few names beginning with J but many with R), then you introduce bias because all names do not have an equal chance of being selected.

Nonprobability samples include those acquired by accident, such as when the first fifty people to leave a clinic are surveyed. Also included are purposive samples for which people are chosen because they "know" the most ("According to the top lawyers. . . ."), or are most typical ("As XYZ votes, so votes the nation. . . . ").

Actually locating the names, addresses, and telephone numbers of survey respondents means getting current and accurate lists that you have a right to use and can afford.

How large should a sample be? For surveys the results of which can affect many people or the findings of which are to be part of research studies that are to contribute knowledge, statistical methods are available to help you sample representatively. When you use statistics, you must be concerned with how confident you are that the sample and population only differ by some specified amount (or sampling error).

When your survey is fashioned to meet specific needs of certain consumers (such as when you survey employees to find out how the department can be improved so that management can plan more efficiently), the sample should be large enough to satisfy the consumer and enable the surveyor to analyze the results appropriately.

How high should a response rate be? As high as possible. If you have used random sampling methods, losing people's responses introduces bias; if you have not, it results in loss of credibility. You can improve the response rate by using survey techniques that have good response rates; plan in advance to replace people who drop out; or prove (afterwards) that the people who responded are like the ones who did not respond in terms of such important factors as age, sex, income, place of residence, education, and the like.

SAMPLE SIZE AND RESPONSE RATE:
WHO AND HOW MANY

When you decide to conduct a survey, you almost always have a fairly good idea of which people you want to include. The trick is to get enough people whose views count. Should you include everyone or just sample some portion of the group?

Suppose you wanted to find out if your neighbors will support a community watch program in which each household would take responsibility for watching at least one other house when the owners were away. Consider also that you define your community as having 1000 homes. Do you need to include all households? If you do, will the watch be more likely to work than otherwise? Here are some questions you should answer.

(1) How quickly are data needed? Suppose a recent increase in house burglaries was the motivation for the survey, and you wanted to get started immediately. If you waited to survey all 1000 homes in your neighborhood, you might be wasting precious time.

(2) What type of survey is planned? If you are going to use a telephone survey or self-administered questionnaire that is dropped in people's mailboxes and returned to a central point in the neighborhood, your survey may take less time than if you plan to interview people in their homes.

(3) What are your resources? If they are limited, you might have to select a survey method such as telephone interviewing rather than home interviewing, because telephoning is a relatively inexpensive way to contact neighbors (especially in areas where local calls can be made at low rates).

(4) How credible will your findings be? If all 1000 homes participated, then you would have no problem arguing that your survey was representative of the neighborhood. If only ten homes participated, you would probably prefer to scrap the survey.

(5) How familiar are you with sampling methods? Sampling methods can be relatively simple or complex. The national polls use very sophisticated techniques that are dependent upon the skills of statisticians and other trained experts.

How do you select a sample? Two groups of methods are available. The first is called probability sampling, while the second is called (of course) nonprobability sampling.

Consider these two cases:

Example: Probability and Nonprobability Sampling

---

(1) A survey was to be conducted to find out how teachers in the Loeb School felt about certain school reforms. All 75 teachers' names were put into a hat, the names were jumbled, and the principal selected 50 from the hat.

(2) A survey was to be conducted to find out how teachers in the Los Hadassah School District felt about certain school reforms. Five teachers were chosen to be interviewed from each of the district's six elementary schools; five were selected from its four intermediate schools; and two were chosen from its one high school. All teachers were selected using the following criteria: They had been teaching in the district for five or more years; they belonged to one of three teachers' associations or unions; they had participated in at least one meeting during the past year on the district's school reforms.

In the first survey, a sample of fifty teachers is chosen from a hat. This type of sampling is called probability sampling because everyone has an equal chance (or probability) of being chosen. More elegant ways of choosing probability samples exist, but the point is that the people who are selected are believed to be just like the people who are not. If you survey a probability sample, you will get an accurate view of the whole group, and in survey terms, your sample will be representative of the general population. A sample drawn in this way is said to be representative.

In the second sample, representativeness of all teachers is not the issue. In fact, the surveyors appeared to want a very special group and chose it by setting up specific criteria for inclusion in the sample.

If you sample at all, you have to decide whether your survey needs to be representative and a probability sample or if a nonprobability sample will be all right.

PROBABILITY SAMPLING METHODS

A probability sample should be a miniature version of the population to which the survey findings are going to be applied. Unfortunately, human beings are notoriously shifty and complex; they are difficult to pin down and classify. As a result, many different methods of probability sampling have been developed to suit different occasions. Three of the most commonly used are:

- simple random sampling
- stratified random sampling
- simple random cluster sampling

Simple Random Sampling

A simple random sample is one in which each person has an equal chance of being selected for participation in a survey.

This is simple random sampling:

Example: Simple Random Sampling

You want to sample 100 people from philanthropic foundations for a survey of the type of grants they sponsor. A total of 400 people can provide this information. You place their names in any order. Then, using a table of random numbers (see the Appendix), you select 100 people.

This is not random sampling:

Example: Not Random Sampling

You want to sample 100 people from philanthropic foundations for a survey of the type of grants they sponsor. A total of 400 people can provide this information. In four areas of the country, you select 25 people who work with philanthropic agencies that annually sponsor at least $2 million in grants.

In this case you have put too many restrictions on who gets selected for your sample for it to be considered random. Here is another example of simple random sampling:

Example: Simple Random Sampling

Two hundred nurses, therapists, and social workers employed by a midwest city signed up for an experimental elderly day-care seminar. The city, however, only had enough money to pay for fifty participants. The seminar director therefore assigned each candidate a number from 001 to 200, and, using a table of random numbers that he found in a statistics textbook, selected fifty names. He did this by moving down columns of three-digit random numbers and taking the first fifty numbers within the range of 001 to 200. (The seminar director also decided that this method was easier than picking numbers from a hat.)

The advantages of simple random sampling are:

- simplest of all sampling methods and easiest to conduct
- most statistical textbooks have easy-to-use tables for drawing a random sample
- many computers can draw a random sample for you

Table A.1 in the Appendix provides a list of random numbers.

The disadvantages of simple random sampling are:

- produces greater errors in the results (greater "standard errors") than do other sampling methods
- cannot be used if you want to break respondents into subgroups or strata (for example, 60 percent male and 40 percent female)

To facilitate simple random sampling for telephone surveys, several procedures (often labeled random digit dialing) have been devised. In one, called the plus-one approach, if the telephone number 454-4297 is selected, the actual number called is one to which one digit has been added to the last number, and thus is 454-4298. This technique helps to make up for the fact that in many areas of the country, particularly in urban areas, people sometimes do not list their telephone numbers and thus are not fair shakes for selection for telephone surveys.

Stratified Random Sampling

In simple random sampling, you choose a subset of respondents at random from a population. In stratified random sampling, you first subdivide the population into subgroups or strata and select a given number of respondents from each stratum to get a sample.

You can, for example, use stratified random sampling to get an equal representation of males and females. You do this by dividing the entire group into subgroups of males and females and then randomly choosing a given number of respondents from each subgroup. This method of sampling can be more precise than simple random sampling because it homogenizes the groups, but only if you choose the strata properly. That is, do not sample men and women unless you are planning to make comparisons between them; you should only plan to make comparisons if you have some reason to believe, in advance, that those comparisons might be meaningful. In a survey of voter preference, for example, if you have some evidence that men and women will vote differently, then it makes sense to be sure that your survey includes a sufficient number of males and females so that you can contrast them. With random sampling alone you might find that by chance you have a survey sample that consists only of men or only of women.

Here is how stratified random sampling works:

Example: Stratified Random Sampling

The University Health Center was considering the adoption of a new program to help young adults lose weight. Before changing programs, the administration commissioned a survey to find out, among other things, how their new program compared with the current one, and how male and female students of different ages

performed in each. Previous experience had suggested that older students appeared to do better in weight reduction programs. The surveyors therefore planned to get a sample of men and women in two age groups: 17 to 22 years and 23 to 28 years and to compare their performance in each of the programs.

About 310 undergraduates signed up for the health center's regular weight reduction program for the winter seminar. Of the 310, 140 were between 17 and 22 years old, and 62 of these were men. Some 170 students were between 23 and 28 years, and 80 of these were men. The surveyors randomly selected 40 persons from each of the four subgroups (male, female, age 17 to 22, and age 23 to 28) and randomly assigned every other student to the new program and the remainder to the old program. The sample looked like this:

University Health Center's Weight Loss Program

	Age 17 to 22 Years		Age 23 to 28 Years		
	Male	Female	Male	Female	Total
Regular program	20	20	20	20	80
New program	20	20	20	20	80
Total	40	40	40	40	160

The advantages of stratified random sampling are that

- it can be more precise than simple random sampling and
- it permits the surveyor to choose a sample that represents the various groups and patterns of characteristics in the desired proportions.

The disadvantages of stratified random sampling are that

- it requires more effort than simple random sampling and
- it often needs a larger sample size than a simple random sample would to produce statistically meaningful results because for each strata or subgroup, you must have at least twenty persons in order to make statistical comparisons meaningful.

If you have difficulty selecting a stratified random sample, keep in mind that the same increase in the precision of the results obtained with stratification can generally be produced by increasing the sample size of a simple random sample (which may be easier to implement).

Simple Random Cluster Sampling

Simple random cluster sampling is used primarily for administrative convenience, not to improve sampling precision. Sometimes random selection of individuals cannot be used. It would, for example, interrupt every hospital ward to choose just a few patients from each ward for a survey. Also, sometimes random selection of individuals can be administratively impossible.

One solution to the problem of using individuals as a sampling unit is to use groups or clusters of respondents. This is the purpose of simple random cluster sampling—to avoid being randomly obtrusive.

In simple random sampling, you randomly select a subset of respondents from all possible individuals who might take part in a survey. Cluster sampling is analogous to random sampling except that groups rather than individuals are assigned randomly. This method presupposes that the population is organized into natural or predefined clusters or groups. Here is how it works:

Example: Simple Random Cluster Sampling

The Community Mental Health Center has 40 separate family counseling groups, each with about 30 participants. The directors noticed a decline in attendance in the last year and decided to try out an experimental program in which each individual would be tested and interviewed separately before beginning therapy. The program was very expensive, and the center's directors could only afford to finance a 150-person program at first.

Randomly selecting individuals from all group members would have created friction and disturbed the integrity of some of the groups. Instead, a simple random cluster sampling plan was used in which five of the 30-member groups—150 people all together—would be randomly selected to take part in the experimental program. Each group would be treated as a cluster. At the end of the six months, the progress of the experimental program would be compared with that of the traditional one.

The advantages of simple random cluster sampling are that it:

- can be used when it is inconvenient or unethical to randomly select individuals
- is administratively simple since no identification of individuals is necessary

The disadvantage of simple random cluster sampling is that it is

- not mathematically efficient

Although in the example you have 150 people in the survey, you only really have five units (the five groups of thirty persons each) to study. Why cannot you study each of the 150 persons individually? When people are in groups—classes, clubs, organizations—they tend to acquire similar characteristics and views at least about the group (if nothing else). Studying each individual in a group would tend to be redundant since one person can be expected to perform like every other.

Narrowing the Margin of Error

Surveying a sample is never a perfect substitute for a survey of everyone in the population. The sample you actually get from random, stratified, or cluster sampling is almost always somewhat different from the population by some margin of error. The trick is to make your sample as accurate as you can by keeping the error small.

You can measure the accuracy of a particular sampling method by computing the standard error (SE) of the mean. To understand how the SE works, consider the following example of simple random sampling.

Example: Computing a Standard Error

Say you have a total of six student nurses; if they are all surveyed their scores are as follows:

Student	Score
1	9
2	8
3	4
4	10
5	9
6	2

Variance = 8.64
Standard Deviation (SD) = 2.94

If you choose as a sample for your survey just two of the students, then there are fifteen possible score combinations you can come up with. In this case, the combinations and their mean scores would look like this:

Sample	Mean Score	Sample	Mean Score
1,2	8.5	2,6	5.0
1,3	6.5	3,4	7.0
1,4	9.5	3,5	6.5
1,5	9.0	3,6	3.0
1,6	5.5	4,5	9.5
2,3	6.0	4,6	6.0
2,4	9.0	5,6	5.5
2,5	8.5		

$\bar{X}$ = 105/15 = 7.0
Standard Error (SE) = 1.79

The mean score for the total population of students is 7.0. Note that only one of the samples of two students produces such a mean. A sample will give you a mean score only approximating the true mean; how exact that approximation is depends on your sample size and how much the population varies. (But remember, a bigger sample does not always mean a better sample.)

In this example, the mean scores for the fifteen samples range from 3.0 to 9.5. The standard deviation of these means—all of which are approximations of the population mean—is the standard error of estimate. In this case, the average of the fifteen means is 7.0, exactly the same as the population average. The SE is 1.79. This tells you that an estimated mean will be on the average ± 1.79 points from the true population mean. As the sample size increases, the SE decreases.

The formula for computing the standard error is as follows:

$$SE = \sqrt{[(N - n)/(N - 1)] \; variance \, / \, n}$$

where N = total population size; n = sample size; and

$$variance = \sum_{i=1}^{N} \frac{(X_i - \bar{X})^2}{N} = \text{variance in the total population}$$

(Note: For more information about the mean, standard deviation, and variance, see Chapter 6.)

As you can see, the standard error is a good indication of how much your sample's responses will mirror the total population from which the sample is drawn. The smaller the standard error, the more confidence you can have that the sample is truly representative.

One somewhat expensive way of improving the sampling error is to increase the sample size. In the preceding example of student nurses, here is the effect of the sample size on the standard error:

sample size	SE
1	2.9
2	1.8
3	1.3
4	.9
5	.6
6	0.0

With a sample of just one nurse, the SE is 2.9 for a mean score of 7.0, and using the total population of six nurses produces no error (of course).

NONPROBABILITY SAMPLING

Nonprobability samples are usually easier to draw than probability samples. But gains in efficiency are often matched with losses in accuracy.

Systematic Sampling

In systematic sampling, you pick a unit, say five, and select every fifth name on a list. If a list contained 10,000 names and the surveyor wanted a sample of 1000, he or she would have to select every tenth name for the sample.

Suppose you have a list of 500 names from which you want to select 100 people. You could select a random number between one and ten. If the number three were chosen, you would begin with the third name on the list and count every fifth name after that. Your sample selection would result in the third name, eighth, thirteenth, and so on until you had 100 names.

There is a danger involved in systematic sampling. Lists of people are sometimes arranged so that certain patterns can be uncovered, and if you use one of these lists, your sample will be subject to a bias imposed by the pattern. Here is an example. Suppose you were sampling classrooms so that you could survey students in order to find out about their attitudes in school. Say also that the classrooms were arranged in this order:

Floor	1:	1a,	1b,	1c.
Floor	2:	2a,	2b,	2c.
Floor	N:	Na,	Nb,	Nc.

Suppose also that you selected every third class starting with 1a. The sample would consist of classrooms 1a, 2a, and so on, to Na. This survey of attitudes to school could be biased if each "a" corresponded to a location within the school that faced the lawn and was quiet, while the "b" and "c" classes faced the sports arena and were noisy.

In considering the use of systematic sampling, carefully examine the list. If you suspect harmful bias, use some other sampling method.

Accidental Samples

An accidental sample is one that you get because people are available. Say you wanted to find out whether the student health service was any good. Your plan is to interview fifty students. If you placed yourself outside the clinic door, you could ask each person as he or she walked out to participate in your survey. When you had finished

interviewing fifty students, you would have conducted your survey with an accidental sample.

The most obvious advantage of an accidental sample is that it is convenient. But it may be a very biased sample. Here are several possible sources of bias:

(1) Students who are willing to be interviewed may be more concerned with their health than others.
(2) Students who use the service at the time your interview is conducted may be going for convenience; sicker students may use the service at night.
(3) Students who talk to you may have a gripe and want to complain.
(4) Students who talk to you may be the most satisfied and want to brag.
(5) Employed students may have access to other health services and use them instead.

Accidental samples are usually unconvincing. If you can prove that the most obvious biases are not present, you raise the level of credibility. But the effort seems hardly worthwhile considering that the same amount of effort might be used to produce a better sample. One way to improve this sample for the student health service survey is to use a systematic plan. For example, you might stand outside the clinic for an entire week during all the hours the clinic is open and survey every tenth student.

Purposive Samples

When you use purposive sampling, you are assuming that with good judgment you can handpick your sample. Here are examples of how purposive sampling is used:

Example: Purposive Sampling

(1) For the past three years, teachers in four of the city's schools have consistently expressed views that are similar to all members of the Teachers' Guild. This year, the guild only surveys teachers in the four schools.

Example: Purposive Sampling

---

(2) A total of 100 deans of law schools, senior partners in large law firms, and judges are surveyed to find out which lawyers they would go to to solve their own legal problems.

(3) Why are some college students liberals and others conservatives? Is it their family background? the region of the country in which they were born? college major? A survey is made of members of the Young Conservative Association and the Young Liberals Society.

The basic problem with purposive sampling is that the judgment of the surveyor may be in error. In the first example, the surveyor is assuming that the teachers' views in four schools will continue to be very similar to the rest of the Guild's. But major changes may have occurred in one or more of the schools since the last survey.

In the second example, the "top" lawyers may provide the services needed by deans, senior law firm partners, and judges. Do they offer needed services to the rest of us?

Finally, in the third example, the fact that the only students who are being surveyed are those who belong to organizations may bias the results.

What is the value of purposive sampling? It makes sense if you can justify your choices. Be careful not to oversell the results by claiming that the people in the sample are definitely special or typical because that claim may not be relevant or even true.

FINDING THE SAMPLE

Once you have decided on a sampling method, you have to locate the individuals who will be in the survey so that you can mail their questionnaires to them or arrange for an interview. Identifying survey respondents means going through lists of people who are thought to share certain characteristics or concerns.

How might you find the names, addresses, and telephone numbers of each of the people in these two samples?

(1) Doctors in California who have performed gallbladder operations within the last three years.
(2) Barton School District's male high school English teachers.

Sample 1's doctors might be located by obtaining lists of names from California's professional medical and surgical societies, the phone book's Yellow Pages, or from medical insurance agencies; the Yellow Pages are free. In any case, you must make sure your sources are up to date.

Sample 2's male high school English teachers might be identified through the school's personnel records or the English Department. However, the records may not be readily available to the public. To obtain them, you might have to go through official procedures—the human subjects clearance outlined at the end of Chapter 3—in which you demonstrate that your purposes are sound and that you will keep all information confidential.

Finding the sample means getting a current and accurate list that you have a right to use and can afford.

HOW LARGE SHOULD YOUR SAMPLE BE?

With Statistical Methods

How do you finally decide how many people to include?

The size of the survey can be decided with statistical precision. This is particularly important for surveys that attempt to make large-scale predictions such as forecasting who will win a local or national election, whether business conditions will improve, and if the market for real estate will change. Using statistical methods to estimate sample size is also critical if the survey is part of a research or evaluation study the findings of which might be compromised if one part of it, say a survey, is done poorly.

Look at this:

The National Agency for Health has organized a series of technical panels to provide up-to-date information on the most appropriate use of relatively new medical and surgical procedures, such as coronary artery bypass graft surgery and organ transplants. One of their concerns is that practicing physicians alter their behavior so that newly introduced procedures are used appropriately. Because of their concern, a study is being sponsored to find out the relationship between the panels' recommendations and how physicians practice. As part of the study, a national survey is being conducted to find out how physicians learn about the recommendations: through medical journals? word-of-mouth? Statistical consultants advised that 2500 doctors were needed for the survey's sample to represent the practice of nine medical specialities in all fifty states.

A major concern in choosing a sample size is that it be large enough so that it will be representative of the population from which it comes. No significant differences should exist between the sample and the population on any important characteristic. You will not find the sample much older than the population, for example, nor will it be sicker, wealthier, more educated, and so on. Also, it will be large enough so that important differences can be found in subgroups such as men and women or Democrats and Republicans.

Suppose you wanted to find out why parents in a particular neighborhood choose to send their children to the local private school rather than public school. Suppose also that you suspected that income had something to do with parents' choice. Using statistical methods would help ensure that you get a large enough number of people so that the pattern or distribution of income in the sample would look reasonably similar to the entire populations'.

Three issues must be considered when using statistical methods to choose a sample size: concern with sampling error, stratification, and your confidence in how representative the sample is.

Sampling Error. Concern with sampling error comes about because some small differences will always exist among samples and between them and the population from which they were drawn. One approach to measuring sampling error is the standard error of the mean. You have to minimize sampling error to maximize the sample's representativeness. Think of the population of parents who are eligible for a survey of reasons for sending children to public or private school. These are people who live in your neighborhood and have children of school age. If the average annual family income is $40,000, then you want to make sure that your sample's average is as close to $40,000 as possible. If you cannot get perfect agreement, how close must you get? You should try to keep the difference or error down to a few percentage points from the average.

Stratification. In stratified sampling, the surveyor draws a sample with a pattern of important characteristics (e.g., age or sex) that is the same as the population's. If 75 percent of parents have incomes over $40,000 a year and 25 percent have incomes below $40,000 a year, you would want to be sure that your sample also has the same distribution of income. One type of stratification is simple random stratified sampling.

Confidence Levels. First, you must consider a level at which you will be confident that your sample is representative. Frequently, the 95 percent confidence level is chosen, meaning that you are anticipating that there is a 95 percent chance that the sample and the population will look alike, and a 5 percent chance that it will not. Sometimes, the stricter level of 99 percent is chosen—at others, the more lenient confidence level of 90 percent.

Consider this:

Example: Using Statistics to Determine Sample Size

You are conducting a survey of families in your neighborhood to find out why some parents send their children to public school, while others choose private school. You suspect annual family income has a strong influence on the choice, and that all parents would send their children to private school if they could afford it (meaning an income of $40,000 or above). A previous survey revealed that about 25 percent of the families have annual incomes below $40,000, while 75 percent have annual incomes above $40,000. You decide to use statistical methods for a sample size. Here is a formula you can use:

$$N = (z/e)^2 (p) (1 - p)$$

where N = sample size;

z = the standard score corresponding to a given confidence level;

"e" = the proportion of sampling error; and

p = estimated proportion or incidence of cases.

By definition, for a 90 percent confidence level, z = 1.65; for 95 percent z = 1.96; and for 99 percent, z = 2.58. Traditionally, an acceptable error level is up to plus or minus .10 (ten percentage points).

In your population, 25 percent of the families have annual incomes below $40,000 and thus, p = .25. Using a confidence level of 95 percent with z = 1.96, and an error level of .10, you would calculate the sample size as follows:

$$N = \left(\frac{1.96}{0.10}\right)^2 \quad 0.25 \quad 0.75$$

$$N = \left(19.6\right)^2 \left(0.1875\right)$$

$$N = \quad 72$$

A sample size of 72 families with annual incomes below $40,000 would create no more than a ± 0.10 sampling error with a confidence level of 95 percent for a population with 25 percent of its families earning less than $40,000 a year and 75 percent earning more.

But not all surveys require statistical methods to obtain a sample size that can be considered reasonable. Look at this:

Example: Determining Sample Size Without Statistics

The Midstate University Medical Center has a permanent staff of 100 doctors in its Department of Medicine. In order to find out how much they know about the National Agency for Health's technical panel's recommendations on medical and surgical procedures, a self-administered questionnaire will be given to each doctor. Then, 50 of them will be called to get additional, more detailed information about their reaction to the agency's panel program. (The purpose of the survey is to have the chairperson of the department and the dean of the medical school plan continuing educational programs.)

The Midstate University Medical Center is concerned with its educational planning process. As long as the dean and chairperson are satisfied that all faculty will be contacted with just half being interviewed, then the sample is large enough. And in surveys the purposes of which fall on the "specific uses" end of the generalizability continuum, the rule is that the size of the sample should be large enough to yield useful data.

RESPONSE RATE

The response rate is the number of people who respond to a survey. It is calculated by dividing the number of completed surveys by the number of surveys that could have been completed. If you tried to interview 100 and 75 completed interviews were obtained, your response rate would be 75 percent. How high should the response rate be? You must try to get it as high as you can. If your sample was chosen statistically, then a low rate introduces error. If it was not, a poor response rate reduces the survey's credibility. If your rate is very low, you must find out if the people who responded are different from the ones who did not. Are they more motivated or sympathetic to the topic of the survey? If so, you cannot rely on their biased responses for valid information.

How can you improve the response rate? Try these suggestions.

(1) Use a technique that usually has a high response rate. Face-to-face interviews produce better results than mailed questionnaires.

(2) Plan in advance to replace nonrespondents. If only half your neighbors have been randomly selected to be included in your original survey of support for a community watch, the other half can serve as replacements. Sometimes it is worth oversampling: select more people than you really intend to use so that you can replace dropouts relatively easily. Do not wait until the survey has begun to replace these dropouts, because it is administratively more complex and you will probably introduce bias.

(3) Prove that the loss of data from nonrespondents does not harm or bias the survey's findings. You might do this by showing that no obvious differences exist among respondents and nonrespondents in such factors as age, education, experience, income, and so on.

5

SURVEY DESIGN
Environmental Control

OVERVIEW

A survey's design is the way in which its environment is controlled. The design variables over which surveyors have control are when the survey is to be given, how often, and the number of groups to be surveyed.

A cross-sectional design provides a portrait of things as they are at a single point in time. A poll of voters' preferences one month before an election and a survey of the income and age of voters in the same election both use cross-sectional designs.

Longitudinal surveys are used to find out about change. Trend designs are longitudinal. When you survey one group of sixth graders in 1980, another group in 1982, and a third group in 1984, you have a trend design. Another longitudinal design is the cohort. If you take a sample of children who were sixth graders in 1984, and in 1985 take another sample from the 1984 group, you are studying cohorts. A third longitudinal design is the panel. When you take 100 children who are sixth graders in 1982 and survey the same 100 in 1984, you have a panel design.

In comparison group survey designs, the groups you survey can be assembled randomly or in some other way, perhaps voluntarily. Random assignment usually makes it easier to draw valid conclusions from survey data. Normative designs take two forms. In the first, two groups are compared, but only one is actually surveyed; the other group, the comparison, consists of data that are already on record. The second type of normative design uses a "model" as a standard for comparison.

A case control design is one in which groups of individuals are chosen because they have (the case) or do not have (the control) the condition being studied, and the groups are compared with respect to existing or past attitudes, habits, beliefs, or demographic factors that are judged to be of relevance to the causes of the condition.

WHAT DESIGNS ARE AVAILABLE?

Survey data can be used to describe the status of things, show change, and make comparisons. You must choose a design that will result in the kind of data you need. The "design" refers to the way in which the survey environment is controlled or organized. The more control you have, the more credible your results will be. The variables over which surveyors have control are as follows: (1) when the survey is to be given (for example, after graduation); (2) how often (for example, once a year for three years); and (3) the number of groups (for example, one, a sample of graduates; or two, all people in Programs A and B).

During sampling, choosing the sample and getting an adequate sample size and response rate are the main issues. When designing a survey, the chief concerns are with when and how often the survey will be given and to how many groups (no matter how the groups were selected or their size).

Look at these five surveys planned by the Have-A-Heart Association.

Example: Surveys with Differing Designs

---

(1) The Have-A-Heart Association offers educational programs to people in the community. In June it is conducting a survey of a random sample of people to find out and describe which programs they prefer.

(2) The Have-A-Heart Association wants to know how much knowledge people acquired in its educational programs. Surveys have been conducted with random selections of participants from programs that were offered in 1983, 1984, and 1985, and the results were compared.

(3) The Have-A-Heart Association has been concerned with monitoring community attitudes toward the role of proper diet in the possible prevention of heart disease. An educational campaign was launched in 1970. Every five years since then, the association has been monitoring attitudes by surveying a different random sample of people who were in the original program. This means that some people are surveyed more than once, while others are not surveyed at all.

(4) The Have-A-Heart Association has been concerned with monitoring community attitudes toward the role of a proper diet in the possible prevention of heart disease. An educational campaign was launched in 1970. Every five years since then, the Association has been monitoring the attitudes of the same 500 people who were in the original program and have volunteered to participate as long as the survey lasts.

(5) The Have-A-Heart Association is considering the merits of two competing six-month programs to prevent heart disease. A survey comparing participants' knowledge and attitudes toward diet and exercise will be conducted at the program's completion from random samples of participants in Programs A and B.

The first survey is to be conducted in June to describe the programs that the community prefers. The design, in which data are collected at one point in time, is called cross-sectional.

The second survey calls for collecting information over a three-year period and comparing each year's results with the others. This is called a longitudinal design, and, specifically, a trend design.

The third survey means that every five years you survey a different random sample of people from the original program. This design is called a cohort.

In the fourth survey, the same group provides respondents for a longitudinal study, and the design is called a panel.

The fifth survey is different in that it calls for comparisons between two programs and requires a comparison group design.

Table 5.1 shows the relationships among the purposes, sampling and design concerns, results, and type of design for the five Have-A-Heart Association surveys.

CROSS-SECTIONAL SURVEY DESIGNS

With this design, data are collected at a single point in time. Think of a cross-sectional survey as a snapshot of a group of people or organizations. Suppose the Have-A-Heart Association wants to know which of its educational programs the community prefers. Consider this question and its answer.

Example: Cross-Sectional Design

Question: If only one program were possible, which would you choose?

Sample: A cross section of 500 people, randomly selected, who attended an educational program this year.

Design: Cross-sectional

Method: Telephone interviews

Answer: Dine-Out wins. Here is proof (using hypothetical data):

TABLE 5a Educational Programs Preferred Most by Men and Women Participants

	Men		Women		Total of Men and Women	
	Number	Percentage	Number	Percentage	Number	Percentage
Dine-Out	168	34	175	35	357	69
Feel Fit	75	15	50	10	97	25
Emergency Care	21	4	11	2	46	6
Totals	264	53	236	47	500	100

TABLE 5.1 Relationships Among Purposes, Sampling and Design Concerns, Results, and Type of Design in Five Surveys Given by the Have-A-Heart Association

The Survey Is to Find Out About:	Concerns of Sampling	Concerns of Design	Its Results	Type of Design
Preference for educational programs	A random sample of program graduates	When conducted: this year	Description of preferences	Cross-sectional
Knowledge acquired from educational programs	Different random samples of graduates	When conducted: 1983, 1984, 1985	Estimate of changes in knowledge	Longitudinal: Trend
Attitude toward diet in prevention of heart disease	Samples of randomly selected and possibly different graduates of the original program	When conducted: 1970, 1975, 1980, 1985	Estimate of changes in attitude	Longitudinal: Cohort
Attitude toward diet in prevention of heart disease	Same sample of 500 program graduates	When conducted: every five years (1970 to 1985)	Estimate of changes in attitude	Longitudinal: Panel
The merits of the program	Randomly selected graduates from program A and graduates from program B	When conducted: Once, when program is completed How many groups: Two (A and B)	Comparison of knowledge and attitudes	Comparison

TABLE 5b Educational Programs Preferred Most by Participants of Different Ages

	21-45 Years		46-65 Years		Over 65 Years		Total	
	Number	Percentage	Number	Percentage	Number	Percentage	Number	Percentage
Dine-Out	99	20	96	19	41	8	236	47
Feel Fit	35	7	37	7	90	18	162	32
Emergency Care	47	9	52	10	3	1	102	21
Totals	181	36	185	37	134	27	500	100

Assuming that a sample of participants has been wisely chosen by a random sampling technique and the right questions have been asked, the tables in the above example reveal that Dine-Out is the winner. This is why:

(1) Regardless of sex or age, Dine-Out is ahead.
(2) More men than women prefer Feel Fit and Emergency Care. But when it comes to Dine-Out, men and women have nearly the same preference.
(3) People over 65 prefer Feel Fit, but there are not so many of them as people in the other two categories.

Of course, you might want to use only Table 5a or just Table 5b to make a point about your survey. But a cross-sectional design that is carefully planned will give you a variety of ways for analyzing and presenting your survey data.

With this program preference data, for example, you might also have considered profession—How do people in business and the professions compare? Does retirement make a difference?—or residence—How do people in one part of the city compare with people in some other part?

Cross-sectional surveys have several advantages. First, they describe things as they are so that people can plan. If they are unhappy with the picture a cross-sectional survey reveals, they can change it. Cross-sectional surveys are also relatively easy to do. They are limited, however, in that if things change rapidly, the survey information will possibly become outdated.

LONGITUDINAL SURVEYS

With longitudinal survey designs, data are collected over time. At least three variations are particularly useful.

Trend Designs

A trend design means surveying a particular group (sixth graders, for example) over time (once a year for three years). Of course, the first group of sixth graders will become seventh graders next year, so you are really sampling different groups of children. You are assuming that the information you need about sixth graders will remain relevant over the three-year period. Look at this example with participants in programs sponsored by the Have-A-Heart Association:

Example: Trend Design

Question: What do participants know about heart disease?

Sample: Random samples of 500 participants attending Dine-Out in 1983, 500 in 1984, and 500 in 1985.

Design: Longitudinal, trend

Method: Self-administered questionnaires distributed and supervised by program instructors.

Answer: In all three years, participants consistently know little about disease prevention, but by 1984 and 1985, they are beginning to learn about diet, and they appear to know the causes of heart disease by 1985.

Proof (using some more hypothetical data) is displayed in the following table.

Participants' Knowledge of Heart Disease (N = 1500)

	Causes of Disease	Nutrition	Prevention
1983	little	little	little
1984	some	some	little
1985	much	some	little

SOURCE: Scores on the Heart Disease Information Scale, Health Survey Foundation, Los Angeles, 1982. (fictitious)

As with cross-sectional studies, you could have analyzed the results of the heart disease knowledge survey by comparing men and women, different age groups, professions, and so on.

Cohort Designs

In cohort designs, you study a particular group over time, but the people in the group may vary. Suppose, for example, you wanted to study cer-

tain people's attitudes toward diet as a means of preventing heart disease after they have participated in a special program sponsored by the Have-A-Heart Association.

You might survey a random sample of the program's participants in 1985, and then, in 1995, choose a second random sample from the 1985 participants and survey them. Although the responses of the second sample might turn out to be entirely different from the first, you would still be describing the attitudes of the participants in 1985.

Think about this example, in which surveyors follow participants from a program given in 1970 to find out about attitudes toward diet and how those attitudes changed over time.

Example: Cohort Design

Question: How have attitudes toward diet changed since 1970?

Sample: A different random sample of participants is surveyed every five years from among the graduates who participated in a special Have-A-Heart Association program in 1970.

Design: Longitudinal, Cohort

Method: Mailed self-administered questionnaires

Answer: In general, attitudes toward diet have improved dramatically since 1970. No relationship was found between sex and attitude, however. In 1970 and 1980, women had poorer attitudes than men, but the situation was reversed in 1975 and 1985. For proof, see the figure below.

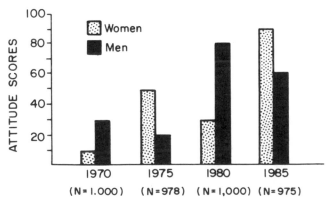

1970 GRADUATES' ATTITUDE TOWARD DIET AS A MEANS OF PREVENTING HEART DISEASE

Source: Attitude toward Diet Inventory," McConnell Publishing, New York, N.Y.: 1965. (fictitious)

As can be seen from the figure, mens' and womens' attitudes fluctuated with time, although they both got better. What happened? Unless you systematically monitor the events that affect the graduates of the 1970 program, you will not be able to tell from the survey results.

The only way to comprehend fully the cause of events is to put together large-scale true experimental studies that conform to scientific methods for gathering reliable and valid evidence. Here is where a survey is truly ineffective.

Panel Designs

Panel designs mean collecting data from the same sample over time. If you were concerned with monitoring attitudes toward diet of graduates of an educational program given in 1970, you would select a sample of participants and follow them and only them throughout the desired time period.

One way to display the results of your data might be as shown in the following example:

Example: Panel Design

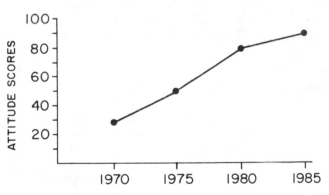

1970 GRADUATES' ATTITUDE TOWARD DIET AS A MEANS OF PREVENTING HEART DISEASE

Source: "Attitude Toward Diet Inventory," McConnell Publishing, New York, N.Y. (fictitious)

COMPARISON GROUP SURVEY DESIGNS: QUASI- AND TRUE EXPERIMENTS

With these designs, people are divided into two or more groups. The classical comparison group design contrasts an "experimental" group with a "placebo" group. Consider this:

(A) A survey is conducted of voters' preference for candidates for the school board. As part of the analysis, the preferences of men and women are then compared.

(B) How do you get people to participate in school board elections? A month before the elections, two groups of volunteers were assembled. The first group was given a television presentation, and the second was given a talk by prominent people in the community. A survey was taken a week after the election to compare the number of people who voted.

Only B uses a comparison group design since the two groups were specifically created for comparison purposes.

Comparison group designs are frequently divided into quasi- and true experimental designs. In quasi-experimental designs, assignment to groups is usually deliberate and not at all random. In true experimental designs, individuals may become members of one group or another: It is mainly a matter of chance. True experiments are the more powerful.

Sometimes longitudinal designs and comparison group designs can be combined. If the various groups included in a comparison group design are each surveyed several times (say every two months or two years), the result is both a longitudinal design and a comparison group design.

Example: A Quasi-Experimental Design

You have been asked to evaluate two programs for the elderly. Eligible participants are assigned to the programs on a first-come, first-served basis, resulting in 60 people in Program 1 and 59 in Program 2. One of the issues addressed by a survey is whether the participants are satisfied with the staff of their program. To answer this question, you ask participants in both groups to complete a questionnaire at the end of three months' treatment. The design for this survey looks like this:

Attitudes Toward Staff of Participants in Two Programs for the Elderly*

Program 1 N = 59	Program 2 N = 60

*Data source: scores on Attitude to Staff Questionnaire.

How valid is the quasi-experimental comparison group design used for the survey of the attitudes of the elderly in two programs toward their staff? Consider these possibilities:

(1) Participants in the two groups may be different from one another at the beginning of the program. For example, older persons may choose one program over the other.
(2) Participants who truly dislike the staff in one of the programs may have dropped out of the programs.

Example: A Quasi-Experimental Comparison Group and a Longitudinal Design

Another question posed for the evaluation of the two programs for the elderly is whether participants have learned about commonly prescribed drugs. To answer this question, participants have been interviewed at three times: at the beginning of the program, at the end

of the first month, and at the end of the first year. This survey design strategy can be depicted as:

Changes in Knowledge of Commonly Prescribed Pharmaceuticals in Two Programs*

Time	Program 1 (N = 60)	Program 2 (N = 59)
Beginning of program		
End of first month		
End of year		

*Data source: interview with participants in each program.

The validity of this design may be threatened if persons with serious health problems are by chance more often assigned to one program over the other or by a different drop out rate.

Example: A True Experimental Comparison Group Design

The government commissioned a survey to determine which of three programs for the elderly was the most effective. Among the concerns was the cost of the programs. A comparison group design was used in which people at the Freda Smith Center were randomly assigned to one of three programs, and the costs of the three programs were compared. Program 1 had 101 people; Program 2, 103; and Program 3, 99.

A Comparison of the Costs of Three Programs for the Elderly* at the Freda Smith Center**

Program 1 (N = 101)	Program 2 (N = 103)	Program 3 (N = 99)

*Participants were randomly assigned to programs.
** Data source: interviews with financial experts and . . . .

This design is an extremely powerful one. Because people were randomly assigned to each program, any sources of change that might compete with the program's impact would affect all three groups equally. However, do remember that although people were assigned randomly to the programs within the Freda Smith Center, other centers may differ, and therefore, the findings from the survey may not be applicable to other places.

Example: A True Experimental Comparison Group Design and a Longitudinal Design

---

Programs 1 and 2 in the Freda Smith Center proved to be equally cost-effective. The government then commissioned a study to determine which program was considered by participants to deliver the better medical care. To make the determination, a comparison group design was selected in which care was assessed from the beginning and end of the program and compared among people in programs 1 and 2. The design was depicted by the following diagram.

A Comparison of the Medical Care Received by Participants in Two Programs for the Elderly*

Time	Program 1 (N = 101)	Program 2 (N = 103)
Beginning of program		
Completion of program		

*Data Source: The ABY Quality of Care Review System: surveys of doctors, nurses, patients

---

This true-experiment and longitudinal design is among the most sophisticated and will enable you to make very sound inferences.

OTHER SURVEY DESIGNS: NORMATIVE AND CASE CONTROL

Two lesser-known survey designs are the normative and case control. Both offer some control over the survey's environment by making use of special comparison groups.

Normative Survey Designs

Normative designs can take two forms. In the first, two groups are compared, but only one is actually surveyed. The second group, the comparison, is represented by data that are already on record from a previous data collection effort. The second type of normative design appoints a "model" and compares another group to it. Look at these:

Example: Normative Design—Data on Record

The self-esteem of participants in Los Angeles's Youth Program was measured using the Esteem Survey, an instrument that had been validated on a national sample of 5000 people. The national sample was used as a norm, because there was no reason to believe that the L.A. group would be different in self-esteem than the nation. Youth Program scores were thus compared to the national sample's.

Example: Normative Design—The Model

Are physicians in a new academic general medicine practice as satisfied with their work as physicians in a ten-year-old practice? The new practice has been structured to achieve the same goals as the older one. To answer the question, physicians in both practices are surveyed and the new is compared to the model, older practice.

Normative data can be based on the activities of other groups or programs. Normative survey designs can be less expensive and time-consuming than are other comparison designs. Remember, your group and the "normal" one may actually differ in important respects and your survey results will then be less than valid. Suppose the participants in the Youth Program in Los Angeles were younger than the national sample, for example. If age and self-esteem were related, with maturity associated with better survey scores, then the Youth Program would have to work harder to be a success. If you use normative designs, be prepared to defend your choice of norm.

Case Control Design

A case control design is one in which groups of individuals are selected because they have (the case) or do not have (the control) the condition being studied, and the groups are compared with respect to existing or past attitudes, habits, beliefs, or demographic factors that are judged to be of relevance to the causes of the condition.

Case control designs are generally used by researchers who are testing a specific hypothesis, for example, that a connection exists between lung cancer and cigarette smoking habits. Sometimes researchers use case control designs primarily to explore and have no hypothesis. A case control design might be used, for example, in a new study to help find out if certain crucial differences existed between people who are prone to headaches and those who are not.

A case control design needs two groups, and so, a major concern is their selection. Ideally, the two groups should be as alike as possible. Their only difference should be that the case has the condition being studied, and the control does not. Most often, case control designs mean selecting a control that is like the case in ways that are strongly suspected to affect the condition. In a study of people with headaches, the control might be matched to the case so it had a similar proportion of males, females, and so on.

The major weakness of case control designs is that the two study groups may not be alike at all no matter how selected or matched because of impossibility of controlling for all characteristics that may affect the condition. Some matching criteria might be incorrect, for example, or others may be excluded. Here is how a survey could be used with a case control design.

Example: Case Control Design

The Medical Clinic randomly selected 100 of its 2500 patients between 21 and 55 years of age who were prone to headaches and 100 who were not. Half the people in each group were male, and half were female. A survey was conducted to find out about the following in relation to each group:

- typical daily activities
- potential sources of stress
- family history and background
- medical history
- diet

6

ANALYZING DATA FROM SURVEYS

OVERVIEW

Analyzing data from surveys means tallying and averaging responses, looking at their relationships, and comparing them—sometimes over time.

A tally or frequency count is a computation of how many people fit into a category (those who are over 55 years of age or have a cold, and so on). They take the form of numbers and percentages.

The mean is the arithmetic average, and it requires summing units and dividing by the number of units you have added together. The median is a kind of average with an equal number of scores above and below it. Because it is in the middle, it is used to describe typical performance. The mode is a score that has a higher frequency than other scores in its vicinity. It, too, is a kind of average since it describes the prevailing view.

Measures of variation (range, variance, and standard deviation) help describe the spread of scores or views.

Commonly used survey data analysis techniques include the following:

(1) descriptive statistics (mean, mode, median, numbers, percentage, range, standard deviations)

(2) correlations (Spearman rank-order, Pearson product-moment)

(3) comparisons (Mann-Whitney U, chi-square, t-test, analysis of variance)

(4) trends (repeated measures analysis of variance, McNemar test)

The appropriate analysis method to use is dependent upon the answers to at least five questions:

(1) How many people are you surveying?

(2) Are you looking for relationships or associations?

(3) Will you be comparing groups?

(4) Will your survey be conducted once or several times?

(5) Are the data recorded as numbers and percentages or scores and averages?

Should your data be analyzed by computer? Very small sets of data (or some types of data from open-ended questions) probably do not need to be. But questionnaires and interviews generate quite a bit of data for analysis. A ten-item questionnaire given to fifty people has 500 bits of information to tally; establishing relationships (say, between men and women) can make the analysis quite complex.

If you use computers, you must learn to code and column your survey forms in advance of analysis. A code is the numerical symbol that represents a questionnaire's response to the computer. The column number is the location of the coded responses. Keep your codes and column numbers in a codebook.

Data that are keypunched onto cards or put on tape should be verified to see that they have been correctly entered.

WHAT IS TYPICAL ANYWAY? SOME COMMONLY USED METHODS FOR ANALYZING SURVEY DATA

The day has arrived. All the self-administered mailed questionnaires or interview forms have been returned. The response rate is high. All the questions and all the forms have been filled out. Now is the time to find out what the survey shows: How many men responded? women? Are there differences between them? Have their views changed? These questions get answered by analyzing the data to obtain tallies or frequency counts of responses and averages, compute relationships, make comparisons, and estimate trends.

Some analysis methods commonly used in surveys are:

(1) *Descriptive Statistics*. These are the most commonly used, and they are the basis for more advanced techniques. Descriptive statistics for surveys include the mean, median, and mode; measures of variation; (range and standard deviation); and number (tallies, frequencies and percentages).

(2) *Correlations*. These statistics show relationships. A high correlation between height and weight, for example, suggests that taller people weigh more. A Spearman rank-order correlation is used with categorical data, those that come from norminal or ordinal scales. It allows you to determine the degree of association or equivalence between two sets of ranks.

Example: Rank-Order Correlation

A class of 50 college students is administered two attitude surveys. The first polls their views on affirmative action, and the second asks about their political preferences. John scores highest among the respondents on one measure, and average on the second; Jane's scores are the fifth and eighth highest; Bill's scores are the fourteenth and thirteenth; and so on. A rank-order correlation coefficient is computed to see if the two surveys agree: Do people who rank high on one also rank high on the other?

Pearson product-moment correlations are used to establish relationships between two sets of continuous data, those obtained form interval ratio scales. Examples:

(A) The relationship between academic achievement, expressed as a grade-point average, and scores on an attitude-to-school survey are correlated.

(B) The relationship between liberal and conservative views (1 = liberal; 10 = conservative) and family income ($5000 to $50,000) are correlated.

(3) *Comparisons*. Several statistical methods are used by surveyors to compare groups. The Mann-Whitney U test enables you to compare two independent groups—classrooms, for instance—using data from categorical responses. You can also use the Mann-Whitney U for continuous data, especially if your sample is small.

Example: Mann-Whitney U Test

Boston Elementary School had ten fourth-grade students with severe hearing impairments. Four of the students were in a special program to teach them to speak more clearly. At the end of one semester, students in a special program were compared with the six students in the traditional program. A special education expert rated each child's ability to speak on a scale from 1 to 20, with 20 representing normal speech. If more students had been available, the surveyor might have chosen the t-test; but after considering the smallness of the sample size, he decided to use the Mann-Whitney U test to compare the two groups.

The chi-square is also used to make comparisons when you have categorical data.

Example: Chi-Square

A comparison was made between sixty imprisoned men's and forty imprisoned women's responses to a survey of their attitudes toward their family. The table for the analysis looked like this:

Attitude	Men	Women	Total
Poor	57	32	89
Good	3	8	11
Total	60	40	100

The t-test allows you to compare the average views of two groups to determine the probability that any differences between them are real and not due to chance. You should have at least twenty cases per group to compare and continuous data.

Example: t-Test

Two hospitals have initiated a gourmet meal plan. Do differences occur in patients' satisfaction between the hospitals as measured by the Satisfaction Scale (10 = much satisfaction and 1 = little satisfaction), and are the differences statistically different?

Group means can also be tested with analysis of variance (ANOVA), and this method lets you compare several groups at the same time. Of necessity, you will need larger samples as you expand the number of comparison groups.

(4) *Trends*. Special forms of t-tests and ANOVAs can be used to measure change over time. A dependent t-test measures change in a single group from time 1 to time 2. A repeated measures analysis of variance can be used to detect changes in one or more groups at two or more times.

With the McNemar test, each person acts as his or her own control, and small samples and categorical data are used. For example, before and after participation in a counseling program, 25 students are surveyed to find out if there is a difference in the number who choose careers in engineering, computer science, and business.

PUTTING THE HORSE IN FRONT OF THE CART: SELECTING ANALYSIS METHODS

The appropriate analysis method for survey data is totally dependent on who is surveyed, the survey's design, and the type of data that are collected. If someone asks, as people sometimes do, "What is the best method for analyzing survey data?" reply with five questions that must be answered first and collectively.

(1) *How Many Are You Surveying?* Answering this question means describing the population or sample. Sample size must be carefully reviewed because some statistical methods (t-tests and ANOVA) depend on relatively larger samples than some other methods such as the Mann-Whitney *U*. Look at these examples.

(A) All 500 teachers in the school district.
(B) A stratified sample of 50 teachers in the school district. The strata or divisions are men and women; and high school, junior high school, and elementary school teachers.
(C) Six teachers in Hart senior high school and five in James senior high school.

Do you have sufficient data to compute more than tallies, averages, and the variation? You would for Example A, but you probably could not for Example C.

What about Example B? Suppose you were surveying a population of teachers of whom about 60 percent were women and 40 percent were men. If you took a sample of fifty, and your stratification method were a success, you could have thirty (sixty percent women × fifty) in one group, and twenty (40 percent × fifty) men in the other. Groups of thirty and twenty are just about large enough for some statistical comparisons (a t-test, for example). If you further subdivided the groups, you could find very few people on whom many techniques of statistical analysis would be meaningful.

Consider this:

| | Teachers | |
	Men	Women
Elementary	2	15
Junior high school	3	10
High school	15	5
Total	20	30

If you wanted to compare men and women teachers in elementary school, you would only have two men and fifteen women for your analysis (although for the total, you have twenty men and thirty women). This leads to the second of the five questions.

(2) *Are You Looking for Relationships or Associations?*

Example: Relationships and Associations

(A) What is the relationship between voters' political views (as expressed on the Political View Survey) and number of years of formal schooling? The Political View Survey gives continuous scores ranging from 10 (liberal) to 100 (conservative).

(B) Can an association be found among high, medium, and low scores on the Political View Survey and high, medium, and low scores on the Authoritarian-Libertarian Inventory?

In the first example, the degree of association between the two variables, political views, and number of years of formal schooling, can be computed by using the Pearson Product-Moment correlation because continuous data are available. For the second example, with ranks of high, medium, and low, the Spearman rank-order correlation would be appropriate.

(3) *Will You Be Comparing Groups?* This question is about design.

Example: Comparing Groups

(A) Fifteen teachers in Hart High School will be compared with twenty in James Senior High.

(B) A total of 100 male and female teachers from the district's high schools, junior high schools, and elementary schools will be surveyed in December and June and compared at both times.

If you are comparing groups, statistical methods such as the Mann–Whitney U, t-test, ANOVA, chi-square, and others can help you decide if any observed differences are due to some real occurrence, or if they result from chance or some other factor.

(4) *Will Your Survey Be Conducted Once or Several Times?* This question is to find out whether the survey design is cross-sectional or longitudinal. It asks if you are looking for descriptions or trends. Here is an example of each:

Example: Looking For Trends

(A) All 500 teachers will be surveyed in December.

(B) A sample of 100 teachers will be surveyed in December and again in June.

If the survey will be conducted several times, you can record your findings by plotting them on a graph. Consider this:

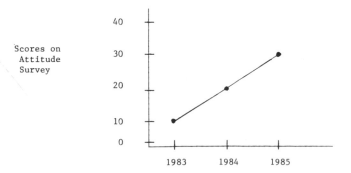

TABLE 6.1 A Comparison of Number of Men and Women Accepted into Law School from Two Coaching Programs

	Coaching Program A (N = 102)	Coaching Program B (N = 206)
Men	50	100
Women	52	106

TABLE 6.2 A Comparison Between Scores of Men and Women in Two Law School from Two Coaching Programs

	Coaching Program A		Coaching Program B	
	$\bar{X}$	SD*	$\bar{X}$	SD*
Men	20.6	2.3	42.8	2.9
Women	15.7	1.4	40.2	2.1

SOURCE: "Attitude Towards Government Survey." (fictitious)
NOTE: Scores can range from 10 = low to 50 = high.
*Standard deviation.

Looking at the graph, scores went up each year by ten points. But is this increase meaningful? As with comparisons, statistical methods, such as the dependent t-test and repeated measures analysis of variance, are available that, if used appropriately, will help you determine meaning over time.

(5) *Are the Data Recorded as Numbers and Percentages or Scores and Averages?* Look at this:

(1) One set of survey data consists of the number and percentage of teachers who agree or disagree with statements about the district's educational policies.
(2) One set of data consists of scores on a measure of attitudes (liberal versus conservative) to various approaches toward education.

Survey data can be in numbers and percentages, (categorical data) or scores that are amenable to the computation of averages (called continuous data). The analytic techniques you would use with each are different. Look at Tables 6.1 and 6.2.

Comparing numbers of people who got accepted into law school from different programs (categorical data) and comparing scores on an attitude inventory (continuous data) require dif-

ferent analysis techniques. (The first comparison might use the chi-square, for example, while the second might rely on analysis of variance.)

A TECHNICAL INTERLUDE

How does the surveyor compute the statistics that describe survey results?

Tallies or Frequency Counts

Consider this:
A survey was conducted of fifty nursery schools receiving support from the city. The following question was asked of each project director.

Example: Preschool Purposes Questionnaire

Following are some possible objectives of preschool education. Circle how important each is in guiding your school's program.

Example: Preschool Purposes Questionnaire

Preschool Education Objectives	(1) Definitely Important	(2) Important	(3) Neutral	(4) Not Important	(5) Definitely Not Important
(1) To encourage creativity through music, dance, art	1	2	3	4	5
(2) To foster academic achievement in reading, math, and other subjects	1	2	3	4	5
(3) To promote good citizenship	1	2	3	4	5
(4) To enhance social and personal development	1	2	3	4	5

A tally or frequency count is a computation of how many people fit into a category (e.g., over 55 years of age; have a cold) or choose a response (e.g., definitely very important, more than three times a week). For the preschool purposes question, you could tally the responses as shown in the following example:

Example: Tallying Questionnaire Responses

Purpose	Number and Percentage of Preschool Directors Choosing This Purpose as Definitely Important	
	N = 50	Percentage
Academic achievement	20	40
Creativity	13	26
Citizenship	11	22
Social and personal development	6	12

Tallies and frequencies take the form of numbers and percents. Sometimes you might want to group the responses together (or, in technical terms, prepare a frequency distribution of grouped responses), as shown in the next example:

Example: Frequency Distribution of the Ratings of Preschool Purposes by Fifty Preschool Directors

Preschool Purpose	Number of Directors Choosing These Ratings		
	Definitely Important or Important	Neutral	Definitely Not Important or Not Important
Academic achievement	40	10	0
Creativity	15	5	30
Citizenship	26	10	5
Social and personal development	7	1	42
Total	88	26	77

Averages: Means, Medians and Modes

The mean, median, and mode are all measures of average or typical performance.

The Mean. The arithmetic average, the mean, requires summing units and dividing by the number of units you have added together. Here are five scores: 50, 30, 24, 10, 6.

The average for these five scores is 50 + 30 + 24 + 10 + 6 divided by 5 = 24.

The formula for the mean is:

$$\mu x = \frac{\Sigma x}{N}$$

μ is the symbol for the mean, and Σ stands for the sum, so Σx means to add all the numerical values such as x and N stands for the number of xs.

Suppose you wanted to compute the average ratings for the four preschool purposes. First you'd have to know how many directors assigned each rating to each purpose (see Table 6.3).

To compute the average rating for each purpose, you would multiply the number of directors who chose each point on the scale times the value

Analyzing Data from Surveys

TABLE 6.3 Ratings of Fifty Preschool Directors

Purpose	(1) Definitely Important	(2) Important	(3) Neutral	(4) Not Important	(5) Definitely Not Important
Academic achievement	26	20	4	0	0
Creativity	13	2	5	20	10
Citizenship	11	24	10	5	0
Social and personal development	6	1	1	30	12

TABLE 6.4 Average Importance Ratings Assigned by Fifty Preschool Directors

Purpose	Rating
Academic achievement	1.56
Citizenship	2.18
Creativity	3.24
Social and personal development	3.82

of the scale. (For creativity, thirteen directors chose a 1, so you would multiply 13 × 1, add the results together [13 × 1] + [2 × 2] + [5 × 3] + [20 × 4] + [10 × 5] and divide by the number of directors: 13 + 4 + 15 + 80 + 50 divided by 50 = 3.24, the average rating for creativity.

In this case, the closer the averages are to 1, the more important the purpose; see Table 6.4.

The Median. The median is the point on a scale that has an equal number of scores above and below it. Another way of putting it is that the median is at the fiftieth percentile. Since the median always falls in the middle, it is used when you want to describe "typical" performance.

Why do you need typical performance? Suppose you had a set of scores like this: 5, 5, 6, 6, 6, 8, 104.

The average is 20, the median is 6. How could this happen? It might if the group you were sampling was divided in its attitude, with most people feeling one way and some feeling much different. It could also happen if you were unable to collect all the data you had planned to, and many of the people with one view were not represented in the responses. Here is how to compute the median if you have an equal number of scores:

(1) Arrange the scores in order of size.

(2) Place the median between the N/2 score and the (N/2) + 1 score (where N equals the number of scores), using the arithmetic average.

Example: Computing the Median for Even Number of Scores

Take these scores: −2, 0, 6, 7, 9, 9

There are six scores so N = 6, with N/2 = 3 and (N/2) + 1 = 4. The third score in order equals 6, and the fourth equals 7, so the median is 6.5.

Take these scores: 2, 4, 5, 8, 9, 11

Again N = 6 so the median is between the third and fourth scores—5 and 8. This time, however, there is a gap of three units between the third and fourth scores. Adding the two scores 5 + 8 and dividing by 2 gives a value of 6.5 for the median.

When a set of data is small and odd in number:

(1) Arrange the scores in order of size.

(2) Place the median at the score that is the (N + 1)/2 from the bottom of the distribution.

Example: Computing the Median for an Odd Number of Scores

Try these: −9, −8, −6, −6, −4, −3, −2, 0, 2

The median of these nine scores is (9 + 1) / 2 or the fifth score, and so the median is −4.

But suppose that in either an even-numbered or odd-numbered set of cases, you have several identical scores at the median or bordering it, as with this set: 3, 6, 7, 8, 8, 8, 9, 9, 10, 12.

When N = 10, as in this case, the median would usually fall between the fifth and sixth score. Calling 8 the median this time will not work because you need five different scores above and five different scores below.

But if you consider a score of 8 as part of a continuum that is evenly spread throughout the interval between 7.5 and 8.5, you can interpolate and come up with an intermediate score.

Think of it this way:

You have three cases (3, 6, 7) until you come to the interval of 7.5 to 8.5, which contains three 8s. Within that interval you will need two more cases to make a total of 5. So, you add two-thirds of the distance or .67 to 7.5, and you get a median of 8.17.

The Mode. The mode is a score (or a point on the score scale) that has a higher frequency than other scores in its vicinity. Look at these scores:

Distribution A		Distribution B	
Score	Frequency	Score	Frequency
34	2	34	0
33	6	33	1
32	8	32	7
31	11	31	11
30	15	30	4
29	18	29	3
28	16	28	7
27	12	27	10
26	8	26	18
25	3	25	23
24	1	24	11
23	0	23	5
	100		100

Distribution A has a single mode of 29, with 18 people getting that score. This distribution is called unimodal. Distribution B has two modes, at 25 and 31, so the distribution is bimodal. (Although the frequency of 11 associated with the score of 31 is the same or lower than that of other scores, the score is a mode because it has a higher frequency than the others near it.)

The mode, with its concentration of scores, describes the prevailing view. You might use the mode when you suspect that you have a group with widely differing characteristics. For example, if you suspect that the reason people social action program C did better than those in program D is because they were economically better off to begin with, you might compare their incomes before they entered each program.

If you find something like this, you could conclude that you are probably right.

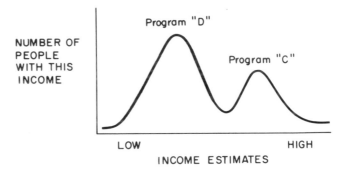

All people in program C are on the high-income part of the scale, while none of those in program D is. Groups C and D together give you a bimodal distribution.

Variation: Range, Variance and Standard Deviation

When you compute an arithmetic average, every number counts. If one or two people have very high or low scores, they can make the average seem artificially higher or lower. Using the median helps, but it too can be misleading. Consider this set of scores: 2, 3, 4, 5, 6, 7, 8.

The mean and median are 5. If you were to change the last two scores to 17 and 18, the median would stay the same at 5, with three cases above and below that score. The mean would rise to 55/7 = 7.86.

TABLE 6.5   Attendance at Sixty Inservice Training Classes by Teachers at Four Schools

School	N	Average Number of Classes	Range
1	50	55	16-60
2	103	54	53-60
3	86	41	15-59
4	117	47.5	15-60

NOTE: N = number of teachers at a school.

If every number counts, it is sometimes important to study the spread of scores—their variation—to shed light on how the mean came to be what it is. Are all the scores near the arithmetic average? Are some very high or very low? Look at Table 6.5.

If you look at the average number of classes attended at the four schools, you find that it is 47.5. Looking further, you see that at some schools, as few as fifteen in-service classes were attended, while at others, all sixty were. In fact, it is hard not to be struck by the range of attendance. At least several inferences can be made because you have access to the range.

(1) Much variation existed in three of the four schools (1, 3, and 4), with some teachers attending many classes and others attending very few.

(2) In only one school (2) did almost everyone attend about the same number of classes as everyone else.

In some cases, variation is considered an asset. A program to train people to think independently or creatively might expect a survey to reveal a variety of perspectives. You also need variation to make comparisons. If everyone performs equally well or shares the same views, you cannot select the best, the strongest, the most liberal or conservative, and so on. In other cases, however, variation is a disappointment because you want everyone to share the same view or achieve a skill at the same level of proficiency. If the district that is sponsoring the in–service training believes its programs are worthwhile, the wide range of attendance would be disappointing.

Another measure of variation is called the variance, and its square root is called the standard deviation. This is a statistical term based on a score's distance from the mean. In fact, the standard deviation is the average distance the average score is from the mean.

The formula for the standard deviation is:

$$SD = \sqrt{\frac{\Sigma(X - \bar{X})^2}{N - 1}}$$

Suppose you had the following scores on the Attitude Toward School survey: 7, 10, 8, 5, 4, 8, 1, 9, 7, 8. Here is how you'd get the standard deviation.

(1) Compute the mean:

$$\bar{X} = \frac{(7 + 10 + 8 + 5 + 4 + 8 + 4 + 9 + 7 + 8)}{10} = \frac{70}{10} = 7$$

(2) Subtract each score (X) from the mean ($\bar{X}$) or $X - \bar{X}$

(3) Square the remainder from step 2 or $(X - \bar{X})^2$

Score	Step 2 $(X - \bar{X})$	Step 3 $(X - \bar{X})^2$
7	$(7 - 7) = 0$	0
10	$(10 - 7) = 3$	9
8	$(8 - 7) = 1$	1
5	$(5 - 7) = -2$	4
4	$(4 - 7) = -3$	9
8	$(8 - 7) = 1$	1
4	$(4 - 7) = -3$	9
9	$(9 - 7) = 2$	4
7	$(7 - 7) = 0$	0
8	$(8 - 7) = 1$	1

(4) Sum up (Σ) all the remainders from Step 3 or $\Sigma (X - \bar{X})^2$

$$\Sigma(X - \bar{X})^2 = 0 + 9 + 1 + 4 + 9 + 1 + 9 + 4 + 0 + 1 = 38$$

(5) Divide the number in Step 4 by N − 1. (N is the number of scores.)

$$\frac{38}{(N-1)} = \frac{38}{9} = 4.22$$

(6) Take the square root of the result of Step 5.

$$\sqrt{4.22} = 2.05$$

Like the range, the standard deviation is a calculation describing the spread of scores. You will often see the standard deviation in tables of data where means are given. Sometimes, instead of the standard deviation, the variance is used. The variance is simply the square of the standard deviation or the result of Step 5 (4.22).

You can only compute the variance and standard deviation on data from interval and ratio scales because they are continuous. Variation in categorical data from nominal and ordinal scales are best expressed in terms of the range only.

Pearson Product-Moment Correlation Coefficient

Correlations measure the relationship between two variables. They are reported within a range of +1 (perfect positive correlation) to −1 (perfect negative correlation).

When high values on one variable occur simultaneously with high values on another, the two variables are said to be positively correlated, and when high values on one variable occur with low values on another, the two variables are said to be negatively correlated.

In mathematical terms, the correlation is the sum of the products of the deviations of each score from the mean divided by N times the product of the two standard deviations. The formula is:

$$r = \frac{\Sigma(X - \bar{X})(Y - \bar{Y})}{N s_x s_y}$$

where r = the correlation, $X - \bar{X}$ is the first set of scores subtracted from its mean, while $Y - \bar{Y}$ is the second set of scores subtracted from its mean; N = number scores in either set; s_x is the standard deviation of the first set of scores; and s_y is the standard deviation of the second.

Consider the following:

A marketing survey for a women's journal asked two questions: How many magazines their readers received from subscriptions each month and their number of years of education. A correlation was computed to see if these two variables were positively associated.

The data from ten respondents are shown below. Note that you definitely should have more than ten respondents for this type of marketing survey. The scores of ten are used here to illustrate how to calculate a Pearson product-moment correlation.

Respondents	Number of Subscriptions (X)	Years of Education (Y)
1	10	12
2	12	14
3	5	7
4	7	9
5	7	10
6	12	15
7	10	13
8	6	8
9	10	12
10	16	18

When you simplify terms, you come up with the following formula and worksheet:

Simplified formula

$$r = \frac{N\Sigma XY - (\Sigma X)(\Sigma Y)}{\sqrt{(N\Sigma X^2 - [\Sigma X]^2)(N\Sigma Y^2 - [\Sigma Y]^2)}}$$

Formula Steps	Calculations
(1) N (number of pairs)	10
(2) ΣX	95
(3) ΣX^2	1003
(4) ΣY	118
(5) ΣY^2	1496
(6) ΣXY	1222
(7) $N\Sigma X^2 - (\Sigma X)^2$	1005
(8) $N\Sigma Y^2 - (\Sigma Y)^2$	1036

(9) Step 7 × Step 8   1041180
(10) $\sqrt{\text{Step } 9}$ 1020.38
(11) $N\Sigma XY \div (\Sigma X)(\Sigma Y)$ 1010
(12) Step 11 ÷ Step 10 = r   .99

The resulting correlation coefficient of .99 suggests a nearly perfect relationship, and so more education is associated with more magazine subscriptions.

Warning: You can use correlations to identify relationships between variables, but you cannot use them to establish causation. A correlation analysis can show that people who have completed many years of schooling usually subscribe to many magazines, but it cannot show that people subscribe because they had many years of schooling.

Note: ΣX^2 means that you first square each score and then you add the squares. The term $(\Sigma X)^2$ means that you first add all the Xs together and then square the sum.

Analysis of Variance

If you want to compare different groups or study changes that take place in the same group from one time to the next, analysis of variance is a method you should consider. Here is how to proceed.

(1) *Take a Careful Look at the Question to Be Sure ANOVA Is Appropriate.* Remember, ANOVA is used to make comparisons among groups or across times. Here are examples of questions that could be answered using one-way analysis of variance:

- *Question 1:* Do patients in the experimental program have different levels of satisfaction than patients in the traditional program?

- *Question 2:* Do experimental patients change their satisfaction pattern from the beginning to the end of the year?

(2) *Decide Which Comparisons to Make and State Your Hypothesis.* Once the questions are posed, you are ready to decide which comparisons you want to make. For example, in Question 1 you will compare persons in the experimental and the traditional programs in terms of their satisfaction.

To evaluate comparisons for ANOVA, you must restate the question as a proposition or hypothesis to be accepted or rejected. You could rephrase Question 1 in two ways.

- *Hypothesis 1:* On the average, patients in the experimental program and patients in the traditional program have different satisfaction levels.

- *Hypothesis 2:* On the average, patients in the experimental program and patients in the traditional program have the same satisfaction levels.

Because of the mathematical structure, ANOVA cannot directly prove that there are differences among groups. It can only prove that they are not the same. To use ANOVA properly, you must test hypotheses about the sameness or equality of behavior and not the differences. For Question 1, for instance, you would have to use Hypothesis 2. This is called the null hypothesis. The null hypothesis for Question 2 is: The experimental patients' satisfaction pattern is the same at the beginning and end of the year.

(3) *Make Sure You Have the Data You Need in the Form You Need.* ANOVA depends on the use of arithmetic averages and standard deviations. You cannot use ANOVA to test a hypothesis about the equality of two groups' behavior unless you have a way to determine their mean performance. This suggests that your survey use interval or ratio scales.

(4) *Test the Hypotheses and Report the Results.* Hypotheses are tested with an F statistic, which is derived mathematically using the ANOVA formulas. In general, if the F statistic resulting from the ANOVA is a small number, then the hypothesis cannot be rejected. For Question 1, a small F value would mean that you could not disprove the hypothesis that experimental and traditional patients' satisfaction levels are the same.

To test hypotheses, first compute means and standard deviations. Apply the ANOVA procedures to these descriptive statistics to get an F statistic. You will find formulas for analysis of variance in standard statistics texts, but canned computer programs are usually available and should probably be used. ANOVA is not a procedure that readily lends itself to hand calculations.

Table A2 in the Appendix contains the F-distribution. This table lists the smallest value that an F-statistic can take in order to reject a hypothesis. These tables provide F values for different degrees of freedom (df) and significance levels (p). Degrees of freedom are the number of independent scores (or observations) entering into the computation of the statistic. The level of significance (p) refers to the probability of falsely rejecting the hypothesis. Surveyors usually use the .05 or .01 significance level, which means that there are either 5 chances in 100 or 1 chance in 100 that the hypothesis will be rejected unintentionally.

The results of a one-way ANOVA frequently are displayed in the following way:

One-Way ANOVA

Source of Variation	Degrees of Freedom (df)	F Value	Level of Significance (p)

The sources of variation column names the hypothesis being tested (e.g., male and female patients' satisfaction rates are the same) and the error term for the analysis (a mathematical result).

The following is a typical report of the use of a one-way ANOVA: It describes the results of a survey used to evaluate a program to enhance the ego strength of young people.

Example: One-Way ANOVA

Program Description: The new Youth Center, unlike the traditional agency for teenagers, has as one of its purposes to provide a range of educational, psychological, medical, and legal services in one place. The two programs are being compared to see how well each has helped the city's youth by, among other things, improving their ego strength.

Step 1: Question—Do Center participants have better ego strength than participants in the traditional program?

Step 2: Comparisons and hypothesis. A comparison design strategy was used for the study in which participants' ego strength was contrasted in the new and traditional programs. Some 96 participants who were eligible for the new Center and the traditional program participated in the evaluation. A random sampling plan was used to assign them to groups so that 48 participants were assigned to each group. The null hypothesis tested by the analysis was: Participants in the new program and the traditional program have the same ego strength.

Step 3: Getting the data. All individuals who participated in the evaluation were given the River's Ego Strength Survey, a standardized measure that was accepted as valid and reliable for adolescents. The measure was administered at the end of six months of a person's participation. The highest possible score on the inventory was 75 points, and the lowest possible score was zero.

Step 4: Test the hypothesis and report results.

Descriptive Statistics

New Program	Traditional Program
$\bar{X}$ = 46.36	$\bar{X}$ = 45.33
SD = 3.46	SD = 3.78
N = 48	N = 48

Source of Variation	Degrees of Freedom (df)	F Value	Level of Significance (p)
New and Traditional Programs	1	3.22	ns (not significant)
Error	94		

The test of the null hypothesis resulted in an F value of 3.22, which is not statistically significant (because the value in the F-statistic table is 3.94 for 1 and 94 degrees of freedom at the .05 level and 6.90 for the .01 level). Consequently, the hypothesis that participants' ego strength in the new and traditional programs is the same cannot be rejected.

This result was recorded in the surveyor's final report in the following way: The analysis was unable to uncover significant differences in average ego strength between teenagers in the center and traditional program. This suggests that the center was not better able to improve ego strength.

TABLE 6.6

| | Respondent Code Number | | | | | | | | | | | |
	1	*2*	*3*	*4*	*5*	*6*	*7*	*8*	*9*	*10*	*11*	*12*
Men	31	34	29	26	32	35	38	34	30	29	32	31
Women	26	24	28	29	30	29	32	26	31	29	32	28

t-Test

The independent t-test is very similar to ANOVA, only, in this case, two groups are being compared. Unlike ANOVA, however, the t-test does lend itself to hand calculations. Here is how:

Suppose twelve men and twelve women were surveyed to learn about their confidence in their local police force. A score of 0 percent indicated no confidence and a score of 100 percent represented total confidence. The survey results were as shown in Table 6.6

If the surveyor wanted to compare men's and women's confidence in the police, a t-test could be used to test the null hypothesis that there was no difference in men's and women's confidence.

The following worksheet could be used to conduct the t-test:

t-Test Worksheet

GROUP	1 (Men)	2 (Women)
$N =$	12	12
$\Sigma X =$	381	344
$\Sigma X^2 =$	12205	9928
$\bar{X} =$	31.75	28.67

(1) Calculation of group variances.

$$s_1^2 = \frac{N_1 \Sigma X_1^2 - (\Sigma X_1)^2}{N_1(N_1 - 1)} = \frac{(12)(12205) - (381)^2}{12(12 - 1)} \quad s_1^2 = \underline{9.84}$$

$$s_2^2 = \frac{N_2 \Sigma X_2^2 - (\Sigma X_2)^2}{N_2(N_2 - 1)} = \frac{(12)(9928) - (344)^2}{12(12 - 1)} \quad s_2^2 = \underline{6.06}$$

(2) Calculation of t-value.

Steps

(1) $\dfrac{(N_1 - 1)s_1^2 + (N_2 - 1)s_2^2}{N_1 + N_2 - 2} = \underline{7.95}$

(2) $\dfrac{N_1 + N_2}{N_1 N_2} = \underline{0.17}$

(3) (Step 1 × Step 2) = $\underline{1.35}$

(4) $\sqrt{\text{Step 3}} = \underline{1.16}$

(5) $X_1 - X_2 = \underline{3.08}$

(6) $t = \dfrac{\text{Step 5}}{\text{Step 4}} = \underline{2.65}$ $\quad df = N_1 + N_2 - 2 = \underline{22}$

(7) Look up t-value in the Appendix (Table A3); $p = \underline{.05}$

If *t*-value at Step 6 exceeds the table value at a specific *p* level, then the null hypothesis (i.e., that the means are equal) can be rejected at that *p* level.

Since the t-value of 2.65 exceeds the value in the Appendix, of 2.074 for df = 22 (Step 6), the surveyor can conclude that there is a statistically significant difference between men and women, with men having more confidence in their local police.

Chi-Square (χ^2) Test (for Two Independent Samples)

To compute the chi-square statistic, the following formula and worksheet might be helpful.

Complete a table like this:

A =	B =	A + B = _____
C =	D =	C + D = _____

A + C = _____ B + D = _____ N = _____

$$\chi^2 = \frac{N[(A \times D) - (B \times C) - N/2]^2}{(A + B)(C + D)(A + C)(B + D)}$$

Steps

(1) (A + B)(C + D)(A + C)(B + D) =

(2) A × D

(3) B × C

(4) Step 2 − Step 3

(5) Step 4 − N/2

(6) (Step 5)^2

(7) N × Step 6

(8) Step 7 ÷ Step 1 = χ^2

To check for significance, use a statistics table like the one in the Appendix. For this 2×2 table, you have one degree of freedom. If the obtained value (Step 8) exceeds the value in the table at a given p (probability) level, then the obtained value is significant at that p level.

Now consider this example:

Example: Chi-Square

MEDEX is a program designed to encourage high school students to pursue careers in health. The school board commissioned an evaluation to see if MEDEX was a success. As part of the evaluation, 210 high school seniors were randomly selected and half received MEDEX and the other half did not. All 210 students were then surveyed at the end of the school year to learn about their vocational preferences. At that time, two of the students in the no-MEDEX group were disqualified from the evaluation when they enrolled in another program similar to MEDEX.

Evaluation Sample	
No MEDEX	*MEDEX*
103	105

The evaluators organized the data into a table and used a chi-square statistic to test whether interest in careers in health was the same in both groups.

Career Preference	No MEDEX	MEDEX	Totals
Other	80	30	110
Health	23	75	98
Totals	103	105	208

To analyze the data, they applied the chi-square worksheet as follows:

Step 1 = 116585700
Step 2 = 6000
Step 3 = 690
Step 4 = 5310
Step 5 = 5206
Step 6 = 27102436
Step 7 = 5637306688
Step 8 = 48.35 = χ^2

Looking up a χ^2 value of 48.35 with one degree of freedom in a table such as Table A4 in the Appendix shows clear statistical significance at the .01 level, suggesting that MEDEX made a difference in encouraging students to consider careers in health.

STATISTICAL SIGNIFICANCE

Suppose you surveyed the attitudes of two groups of students, one of which was in an experimental reading program. Also suppose that the experimental group's scores were much poorer than the other group's, say by ten points. Could the relatively poorer scores be due to chance or was the new reading program responsible? Anything that is unlikely to happen by chance can be called statistically significant. How much of a difference between the two groups is necessary before you can eliminate chance as the motivation?

To determine statistical significance, you must rely on sampling theory. For example, what is the probability that two random samples of students from the same population would produce mean scores that differ by as much as, say, ten points?

Suppose you decide that a chance happening of one time in 100 is an acceptable risk. This predefined probability (p < .01) is called the level of significance. If the differences you observed would occur no more than one out of 100 times, you can reject the null hypothesis of no difference between groups.

Surveyors usually use the .05 or .01 significance level, meaning that the observed difference in the experimental and traditional programs would be considered statistically significant if the difference of 10 points would occur by chance (assuming the two groups are random samples from the same population) only 5 times in 100 or 1 time in 100.

Understanding Type I and Type II Errors

In testing statistical hypotheses, you must establish rules that determine when you will accept or reject a null hypothesis. It is traditional to use a null hypothesis in which no differences between groups are expected.

Take, for example, a statistical test of an experimental (A) and control (B) reading program, where the null hypothesis is that the mean reading scores for both groups are equal ($H_O : \bar{X}_A = \bar{X}_B$), and the alternate hypothesis is that the mean score for the experimental group is higher ($H_I : \bar{X}_A > \bar{X}_B$).

When you apply a statistical test (such as the t-test) to the data, you do not expect to find "zero differences" in mean scores between the two groups. Instead, the real question is whether the differences are so small that they could have occurred simply by chance. When you select two random samples from the same population, you can expect their mean scores to be close, but not exactly the same.

It is up to you to decide how far apart the scores must be before you are satisfied that the difference is not just an accident. You could choose .10, .05, or .01 as the level of significance, depending on the amount of error you are willing to tolerate in rejecting the null hypothesis.

If you select the .05 level of significance, then about 5 times in 100 you will reject the null hypothesis when it is, in fact, correct. This happens because you are comparing two random samples from the same population, and the probability that they will differ by chance alone is 5 percent ($p < .05$). This situation is known as a Type I error. It is the probability of rejecting the null hypothesis when it is true.

If the level of significance is .01, then the probability of a Type I error is only 1 in 100, or 1 percent. You can select a level of significance that would virtually eliminate the chance of a Type I error, but there are serious consequences. The less likely you are to make a Type I error, the more likely you are to make a Type II error.

A Type II error is when you accept a null hypothesis that is, in fact, incorrect. In that case, the difference between the two groups' mean scores does not fall within the rejection region (say $p < .05$). But in reality, the groups are not alike and the experimental treatment is better (the alternative hypothesis is true).

The power of a statistical test is the probability of correctly rejecting the null hypothesis. Mathematically, power is equal to Type I minus Type II error. From that formula, you can see that Type I errors, Type II errors, and power are interrelated. As the probability of making a Type I error goes down, the probability of making a Type II error goes up, but the power of the statistical test goes down.

This means you have to weigh the consequences and decide in advance which risk to take. Is it better to risk declaring the experimental group the victor when there is actually no difference between them (a Type I error); or is it better to risk saying there is no difference when the experimental group is really better (a Type II error)?

Since statistically significant results seem to be regarded as a research "finding" more often than insignificant results, Type I errors are more likely to find their way into print.

CRACKING THE CODE

A code is a numerical symbol that is used to represent responses to survey questions. Codes are the link between your data and the computer. For the question, When did you stop smoking? the codes are 1, 2, and 3.

(1) less than six months ago
(2) more than six months but less than one year ago   _4_
(3) more than one year ago

The codes will be put on cards or on tape as the first step in the analytic process. The number 4, set off to the right, describes where on a computer card or file the response is to be placed (column 4).

When should you use computers? If your survey consists of only a few items, a small sample of people, and a simple analysis, it is possible that you could just use a hand calculator. Suppose you were to analyze the results of a three-item survey of reading habits and that you had fifty completed questionnaires. Here is the questionnaire:

Example: Sample Questionnaire

---

(1) What is your age?   _6_
   (a) under 21 years
   (b) between 21 and 45 years
   (c) between 46 and 65 years
   (d) over 65 years

(2) In the past month, how many mystery books have you read?   _7_
   (a) none
   (b) one or two
   (c) more than two

Example: Sample Questionnaire

---

(3) When you travel by plane for one hour or more, how often do you take each of the following to read?	(1) almost never	(2) some-times	(3) usu-ally	(4) almost always	
(a) newsmagazine	1	2	3	4	8
(b) newspaper	1	2	3	4	9
(c) novel	1	2	3	4	10
(d) nonfiction book	1	2	3	4	11
(e) other, please name _____	1	2	3	4	12

The analyses you might perform using just the questionnaire results could consist of:

(1) Computing frequencies, that is, the number and percentage of people in each age category who have responded to the survey; the number and percentage of people who have read no mystery books, one or two, and more than two; and the number and percentage of people who almost never read newsmagazines on planes and those who read them sometimes, usually, or almost always; the number and percentage of people who almost always read newspapers, sometimes read them, and so on for all categories of reading matter at each point on the scale.

(2) Determining relationships, that is, to enable you to study if associations exist between how old people are and the number of mystery books they have read in the past month and if associations also exist between age and type of reading matter taken on plane trips of one hour or more.

Although computing the frequencies and relationships by hand for this relatively simple, three-item questionnaire and modest sample is obviously not an insurmountable task, it is clearly time-consuming. The analysis could become even more difficult quite easily. Suppose that half the respondents to the survey of reading habits were male and half were female and that the analysis was to compare reading habits of men and women of different ages. You would need to complete a tally sheet such as the one shown in Figure 6.1 before you could make the comparison.

As you can see, there are at least 160 "cells" in which numbers and percentages must be recorded (there could be more if the "other" category produced an additional, important response).

The analysis could be extremely arduous if more questions were added, if the sample were larger, if two totally different groups' responses were to be compared, or if the same group's responses to the survey were to be compared longitudinally. When the analysis gets out of hand, turn it over to the computer.

Coding the Questionnaire: The Code Book. The data from the survey are given to the computer by means of the codes assigned to each response to a question. So, if you use a computer, you must assign a code to each piece of information you want analyzed. You must also tell the computer where to put the coded response. The location is called a column, since, historically, data have been put on IBM cards with vertical columns. Data are stored on cards by punching holes (using a keypunch machine) within the columns. Each vertical column is divided into twelve spaces, just ten of which are numbered: 0, 1, 2, 3, 4, 5, 6, 7, 8, and 9. Even if you use disk files and store your data on tape, you will still be using the term "column A" to describe one location of a response. IBM cards have eighty columns. Data recorded on tapes are not restrained by this number.

To help you ensure the accuracy and completeness of your survey's codes, it is often useful to prepare a codebook before any data are collected. Look at this codebook for the survey of reading habits.

Example: Reading Habits Survey—Codebook

Column	Item Number	Description
1-4		Respondent Identification Number
5		Card Number
6	(1)	Age
		1. Under 21 years
		2. Between 21 and 45 years
		3. Between 46 and 65 years
		4. Over 65 years
		9. No answer
7	(2)	Number of mystery books read in past
		1. None
		2. One or two
		3. More than two
		9. No answer

How Often Types of Reading Material Are Taken	Men (N = 25)								Women (N = 25)							
	Under 21		21-45		46-65		Over 65		Under 21		21-45		46-65		Over 65	
	N	%	N	%	N	%	N	%	N	%	N	%	N	%	N	%
News magazine																
almost never																
sometimes																
usually																
almost always																
Newspaper																
almost never																
sometimes																
usually																
almost always																
Novel																
almost never																
sometimes																
usually																
almost always																
Nonfiction book																
almost never																
sometimes																
usually																
almost always																
Other																
almost never																
sometimes																
usually																
almost always																

Figure 6.1 Tally Sheet for Comparing How Often Men and Women of Differing Ages Take Different Types of Reading Material When They Fly on Planes for One or More Hours

8   (3a) Frequency with which newsmagazines are taken on plane trips of one hour or more
   1. Almost never
   2. Sometimes
   3. Usually
   4. Almost always
   9. No answer

9   (3b) Frequency with which newspapers are taken on plane trips of one hour or more
   1. Almost never
   2. Sometimes
   3. Usually

   4. Almost always
   9. No answer

⋮   ⋮

11   (3d) Frequency with which nonfiction books are taken on plane trips of one hour or more
   1. Almost never
   2. Sometimes
   3. Usually
   4. Almost always
   9. No answer

79-80   _____

             _____

The codebook contains:

- The numbers of the columns in which each response will be located. A single-digit response (e.g., just one choice) is allocated just one column, while a response with several digits (e.g., the identification number) is alloted several columns.
- The survey item numbers.
- A summary of the content of the item and all possible responses (including no answer).

Looking at the codebook, you know that if you could read the completed computer cards for this survey of reading habits, column 6 of this card would contain each respondent's age, in the form of a punch of 1, 2, 3, 4, or 9. If you use computer cards and you collect data that occupies more than eighty columns, you will need more than one card.

A carefully constructed codebook is the best guide to an accurately coded questionnaire and it should be prepared before coding the survey forms. The survey forms should be coded next and the column numbers placed on them before data are collected. Make sure the column numbers are distinct from item and response numbers. If necessary, head column numbers "For Office Use Only." Check that the codebook and survey forms match perfectly. But remember, the codebook is not just a check on the questionnaire; it can also be used as part of the official record of the survey. It can be extremely useful if, in the future, you should want to do additional analyses. Suppose your survey reveals significant differences in reading habits between men and women. If you were later asked to explore those differences by seeing whether age had anything to do with them (say, you suspected that younger girls and boys would be quite different from everyone else), a quick look at the codebook would tell you what you specifically need to tell the computer just for this specific, additional analysis, namely, that you need the information columns in 6, 7, 8, and so on.

Here are some guidelines for constructing a codebook and coding your questionnaires.

(1) Complete the codebook and precode and put columns on your questionnaire before the survey is administered.

(2) Have the codebook and questionnaire reviewed by at least one other person to make sure you have:
- Coded accurately and completely. Do not forget to include a "no answer" category in the codebook.
- Kept all the responses mutually exclusive.

How would you code this?

Which of the following organizations do you belong to? (Circle all that apply)

(1) American Cancer Society
(2) American Lung Association
(3) American Heart Associate
(4) Girl Scouts of America
(5) Boy Scouts of America

The easiest way would be to rewrite the question like this:

---

15) Circle if you belong to any of the following organizations:

Organization	Belong? (1) Yes (2) No		For Office Use Only
(a) American Cancer Society	1	2	10
(b) American Lung Association	1	2	11
(c) American Heart Associate	1	2	12
(d) Girl Scouts of America	1	2	13
(e) Boy Scouts of America	1	2	14

Notice that you ask about each organization individually. Because of this, each becomes like a separate survey item with separate codes and column numbers in the codebook. The codebook for the question could look like this:

Codebook for Organizational Affiliation

Column	Item No.	Description
10	(13a)	American Cancer Association
		1. Yes
		2. No
		3. No response
11	(13b)	American Lung Society
.		1. Yes
.		2. No
.		3. No response
:	:	:
:		:
14	(13e)	Boy Scouts of America
		1. Yes
		2. No
		3. No response

Housekeeping: Verifying and Cleaning the Data. Survey data that have been keypunched onto computer cards should be verified. The "verifier" looks like the keypunch machine, but instead of being used to punch holes, its purpose is to read punches. The person responsible for verification places the punched cards into the verifier and repunches. When the new and previous punches agree, the card advances to the next column. If the two disagree, a light appears, the machine stops, and the next step is to correct the data.

You must always make sure your data are "clean." This means determining if the data on the cards (or tape) are accurate. Consider this:

A survey was conducted of people's attitudes toward religion. A total of 100 people were randomly sampled from high-, medium-, and low-income neighborhoods. Of these, 91 completed interviews were available. The interview data were placed on computer cards and verified. As part of the analysis, men and women were to be compared to see if they differed in terms of their church or synagogue attendance. A preliminary review of the sample size revealed 62 women and 45 men, for a total of 107 people. The surveyor reasoned that the data from some questionnaires had been entered more than once.

Data are cleaned by having the computer do a trial run. If you ask for descriptive statistics, say frequencies, you can compare the sample size with the number of responses to each question. If you find error you can fix them either by going back to the original questionnaires and seeing which responses were omitted or by eliminating the question entirely.

7

PRESENTING THE SURVEY RESULTS

OVERVIEW

Several techniques are available for presenting survey data clearly. These include reproducing a summarized version of the questionnaire and its responses, tables, pie diagrams, bar and line graphs, and pictures. Each has stringent rules that help make the presentation fair and clear.

How do you select among presentation methods? Make sure you can present your data accurately so that one- or two-point differences (on line graphs, for example) do not seem to be more than they really are. Consider what is expected and conventional. Most research and evaluation studies are expected to have tables no matter what information collection method is used. Think about your ability and resources. Some people are very skilled at producing visual aids; others are less so. Visual aids—graphs and pies—may cost more to prepare than other presentation techniques. Use electronic printers to help with tables and graphs when possible.

Survey information is sometimes given in the form of a written report. A written report should include an abstract and summary. When appropriate, consider having a table of contents, list of tables and figures, a glossary of terms, and sections that describe the survey's purposes, methods (type of survey, sample items or the whole instrument, logistics, validity and reliability information, sampling methods, designs) and findings. Describe any methodological or other limitations such as failure to achieve an expected response rate, one or two badly worded questions, one or two unsuccessful interviews, and the like.

To write clearly, use standard English and define your terms. Use the active voice, avoid too many prepositional phrases, and try a readability formula.

For oral presentations, you must be selective. Use visual aids such as handouts of tables, slides, and transparencies.

Survey results can be shown on the survey form itself, in tables, graphs, and pictures.

REPRODUCING THE QUESTIONNAIRE

You summarize each question along with everything else that might have been on the survey or response form (but do not include coding instructions and other "For Office Use Only" directions). When possible, set the results off in some way.

Presentations in which the questionnaire is reproduced must always be accompanied by explanations. Here is what you cover:

(1) type of survey (interviews, self-administered questionnaires, and so on)
(2) date of survey
(3) sample size and response rate
(4) other explanations (How sample size was selected, whether the response rate is adequate, whether the survey is reliable or valid.)

Example: Reproducing the Questionnaire

Analysis Results (in percentages) of a Survey of
the Choice of School Board Candidate Joan Smith
(June 13, 1985)

	Men	Women	Total
Opinion of Joan Smith			
favorable opinion	23	27	25
unfavorable opinion	11	8	10
undecided	8	14	11
haven't heard enough	56	51	53
don't know	2	1	1
Believe she was chosen because			
best candidate	24	21	22
of pressure	58	62	60
both reasons or other	8	6	7
don't know	11	11	11
Feelings about the choice			
excited	13	22	18
all right	62	54	58
bad idea	20	18	19
don't know	6	6	6

Explanation: How the Survey Was Taken

The *Short View Times* survey of school board candidates is based on a telephone interview conducted on June 13 with 100 people who were randomly selected from the voters' list. We are 90 percent confident that the opinions expressed are within ten percentage points of the opinions we would get had we surveyed all eligible school board voters.

USING TABLES

Tables have at least two major purposes: to provide surveyors with a check on the information they will be obtaining and to provide data to survey users in a convenient form. Consider this: The Family Planning Clinic was distributing a self-administered questionnaire to find out how its female patrons learned about birth control. Many planning counselors suspected that a connection would be found between a patron's educational background and how she obtained birth control information. When putting the survey together, the surveyor created a table outline that looked like that shown here as Table 7.1.

After drafting the questionnaire, the surveyor checked to see that he had included a question on patron's educational background and on how birth control information was obtained. Before the questionnaire was distributed, he checked to see that he had covered all relevant sources of birth control information and that the educational background categories were appropriate. The counselors recommended adding magazines and television to the "How birth control knowledge was obtained" category, and these were included in the questionnaire. The results were as shown in Table 7.2

Educational background and how birth control knowledge was obtained appeared to be connected, confirming the counselor's suspicion. Television was a source of knowledge only for the sample of grade school graduates; the major source for college graduates was a doctor or other health professional. It should be noted that word of mouth accounted for knowledge of the largest percentage of female patrons regardless of their education.

Tables: What They Look Like

Survey reports practically always have tables. Their purpose is to describe respondents and their environment, show relationships, and describe changes and combinations of relationships and changes. Their contents include the number of respondents, the groups being compared, the times for observing change, and the results of the survey.

TABLE 7.1

How Birth Control Knowledge Was Obtained	Educational Background			
	Grade School	Junior High	High School	College
Word of mouth				
Doctor or other health professional				
Written educational material				

TABLE 7.2

	Educational Background			
How Birth Control Knowledge Was Obtained	Grade School (N = 25) %	Junior High (N = 30) %	High School (N = 26) %	College (N = 20) %
Word of mouth	60	65	50	30
Doctor or other health professional	1	5	20	50
School	5	15	15	10
Written educational materials	1	5	5	10
Magazine	1	1	0	0
Television	32	0	0	0

Example: Table Used to Describe Respondents

Symptoms of Illness Reported by 42 Patients in June 1985

Symptoms	Number	Percentage
Dizziness	26	62
Weakness	25	60
Headache	24	57
Nausea	23	55
Abdominal pain	20	40
Chills	19	45
Faintness	16	38
Eye pain	14	33
Extremity shaking	13	31
Hyperventilation	12	29
Collapse	12	29
Dysphea	10	24
Loss of consciousness	9	21
Paresthesias	8	19
Chest pain	6	14

SOURCE: Telephone interviews. (fictitious)

Example: Tables that Show Relationships

Comparison of Social Workers' and Administrators' Perceptions of What the Center Does Best

Center Does This Best	Social Workers (N = 64)		Administrators[a] (N = 11)	
	Number	Percentage	Number	Percentage
Provides constructive atmosphere for development of personality	33	51.6	4	36.4
Gives comprehensive care[b]	36	56.3	6	54.5
Cares for client's health	1	1.6	2	18.2
Teaches specific skills	1	1.6	1	9.1

SOURCE: Mailed self-administered questionnaires, April 1984. (fictitious)
a. Administrators include only personnel who perform supervisory and clerical tasks.
b. Comprehensive care means more than one service to each patient.

Males' and Females' Views on Confidentiality of Services

Want Confidentiality?	Male		Female		Total	
	Number	Percentage	Number	Percentage	Number	Percentage
Yes	171	49.4	711	70.3	882	65.0
No	34	9.8	59	5.8	93	6.9
Don't know/ no opinion	141	40.8	241	23.8	382	28.2
Total	346	25.5	1011	74.5	1357	100.1*

SOURCE: Self-administered questionnaire, February 1984. (fictitious)
NOTE: Males and females differed significantly: chi-square = 49.52; df = 2; p < .01.
*Total is more than 100 due to rounding.

Example: Table that Shows Changes

Benefit Received from Participants in Teen Center

Benefit	Interview I (N = 347) Number	Interview I (N = 347) Percentage	Interview II (N = 210) Number	Interview II (N = 210) Percentage
Increased self-confidence	119	34.3	82	39.1
Medical services	74	21.3	43	20.5
Job skills	53	15.3	31	14.8
New friends	49	14.1	24	11.4
Place to go where people care	33	9.5	13	6.2
Recreational activities	25	7.2	25	11.9
Social service assistance	8	2.3	1	0.5

SOURCE: Face-to-face interviews given at the Teen Center. Interview I took place in July 1984; Interview II, July 1985. (fictitious)

Example: Tables that Show Relationships and Changes

Comparison of One Year's Changes in Black and White Youths' Self-Confidence Levels (in percentages)

Level of Confidence	Black Youth 1983 (N = 128)	Black Youth 1984 (N = 49)	White Youth 1983 (N = 104)	White Youth 1984 (N = 212)
High	0	70	0	69
Medium	57	28	57	31
Low	43	2	43	0

SOURCE: *The LMN Self Confidence Scale* (New York: OPQR Press, 1980). (fictitious)

Comparison of One Year's Changes in Black and White Youths' Self-Confidence Levels (in percentages)

Level of Confidence	1983 Black (N = 128)	1983 White (N = 49)	1984 Black (N = 104)	1984 White (N = 212)
High	0	0	70	69
Medium	57	57	28	31
Low	43	43	2	0

SOURCE: *The LMN Self Confidence Scale* (New York: OPQR Press, 1980). (fictitious)

Some Table Preparation Rules

(1) Tables display columns and rows of numbers, percentages, and scores. You must decide how many columns and rows you can include and still keep the table readable.

(2) Each table should have a title that summarizes its purpose and content. In surveys, the purposes of data in tables are to describe respondents and their environment (for example, symptoms of illness), show relationships (such as social workers versus administrators or males' and females' views on confidentiality), describe changes (such as changes in benefits), and document changes in relationships (such as improvement in self-confidence).

(3) When the source of a table's data is not immediately obvious, it should be given below the rule at the bottom of the table.

(4) When you use a term in a table in a different way from usual, define it. Set off definitions with characters such as asterisks and daggers or superscripted letters.

(5) If you have any additional information to help with an interpretation of the data, such as statistical significance, place it after the body of the table.

(6) Select a table format and use it consistently. The tables in the above examples use captions in which the first letter of each word (except prepositions and articles) is capitalized, as are column headings; two horizontal rules appear after the caption, one horizontal rule appears after the heading, and the table is closed with one horizontal rule. For the responses, capitalize just the first letter of the first word (see the examples).

(7) Present your data in some logical order. One commonly used order is from most frequent to least frequent, although showing data the other way around may also be appropriate. The last two example tables above classify data as being high, medium, and low—categories defined by the survey instrument.

(8) Make sure you include the sample size, and differentiate clearly between numbers of people or responses and percentages.

DRAWING PIE DIAGRAMS

Pies show visually what proportion of the whole each response category occupies. Suppose you were conducting a survey of eighty libraries users' needs and wanted to distinguish the needs of people of different ages. Suppose also that you found that forty respondents were relatively young, say between 18 and 25 years of age, while only ten were between 25 and 35, with the remaining thirty people over 45. You could describe your findings effectively by presenting them this way:

Example: Pie Diagrams

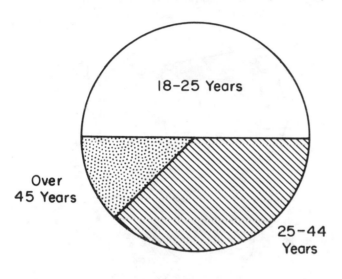

The key to an accurate pie diagram is to draw it to scale. You must calculate the proportion of the whole each response category represents, and draw a slice that reflects just that ratio. In the pie diagram of library users, forty of the eighty people (or one-half) were between 18 and 25 years of age; the diagram has half the area of the pie devoted to these people. Ten of the respondents (one-eighth) were between 25 and 44 years, and 30 (three-eighths) were over 45 years; thus, one-eighth and three-eighths of the pie represent those groups.

Keep the slices to no more than about six, or the pie will get too cluttered.

USING BAR GRAPHS

Bar graphs are commonly used to display survey data because they provide an overview of several kinds of information at one glance. Look at this graph of changes in attitudes toward school between boys and girls from 1965 through 1985.

Example: Bar Graphs

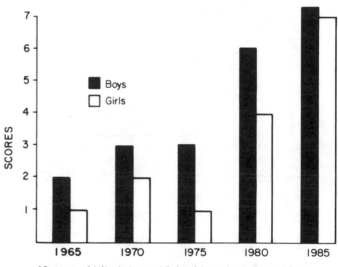

The bar graph enables you to compare boys and girls and to discern trends over time. By just looking, you can see that, in general, attitudes for both improved over time and that girls' scores were consistently lower.

Bar graphs should always have a title, a key to the bars, an explanation of scores, and the source of information.

USING LINE GRAPHS

Line graphs are drawings that allow you to compare groups, show trends, and discern patterns. Be careful not to oversell and make a one-point score look like a major trend (unless it is).

Look at the data previously shown in the first bar graph, showing boys' and girls' changing attitudes toward school.

Example: Line Graphs

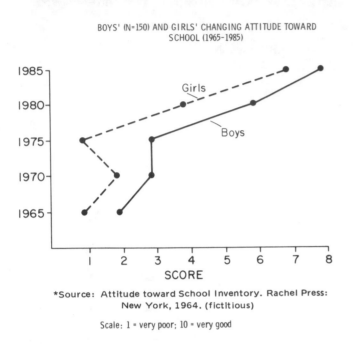

BOYS' (N=150) AND GIRLS' CHANGING ATTITUDE TOWARD SCHOOL (1965-1985)

*Source: Attitude toward School Inventory. Rachel Press: New York, 1964. (fictitious)

Scale: 1 = very poor; 10 = very good

As can be seen, in addition to illustrating that boys' and girls' attitudes improved with time, and that girls were consistently lower, you can compare patterns of responses. In this case, they look somewhat similar. Here are some rules for using line graphs.

(1) Create the Y-axis, which is the vertical one, about three-fourths the length of the X-axis, the horizontal one, or equally as long.

(2) When using percentages or frequencies (number of people with a score of N, or percentage of people over 65 in the sample), use the Y-axis and begin with zero. Scores and other data go on the X-axis and can begin at any convenient point. If a functional status survey is scored on a scale of 1 (much disability) to 10 (little disability) and no one has scores of 1 through 5, you can begin at 6.

(3) Make sure that equal numeric differences are represented by equal physical differences on all scales.

(4) Label the graph to include titles, scales, source of data, and give keys to lines or symbols.

(5) Keep graphs simple.

DRAWING PICTURES

Pictures that accurately display survey data are difficult to create. At the same time, pictures may be helpful in getting your point across. Suppose you are surveying your neighborhood to see how much support there is for a recreational park. Your results might take this form.

Example: Pictures for Displaying Survey Results

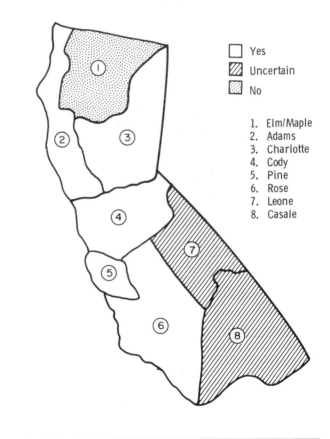

GREEN CITY NEIGHBORHOOD SURVEY: SUPPORT FOR A RECREATIONAL PARK (JULY, 1985)

☐ Yes
▨ Uncertain
▧ No

1. Elm/Maple
2. Adams
3. Charlotte
4. Cody
5. Pine
6. Rose
7. Leone
8. Casale

Here is an explanation of the picture. Green City neighborhood residents were surveyed to find out about their support for a new recreational park. There are eight community neighborhood associations in Green City and each was responsible for administering a questionnaire. Each association created its own rules for coming to consensus. In all, there were 525 completed questionnaires, an overall response rate of 62 percent. The lowest response came from the Elm/Maple Association, which was strongly against a new park. Of the eight associations, five supported the park (Adams, Charlotte, Cody, Pine, and Rose associations); two were uncertain (Leone and Casale); and Elm/Maple was against.

SELECTING SURVEY SUMMARY DISPLAYS

How do you decide whether questionnaire reproduction, tables, graphs or pictures are best? Here are some criteria.

(1) *Accuracy.* A major criterion should be the accuracy with which data can be communicated. Look at this:

Score	Number of People With Score
1	2
2	1
3	3
4	4
5	5
6	4
Total	19

Here are three ways to plot the scores. Which is most accurate?

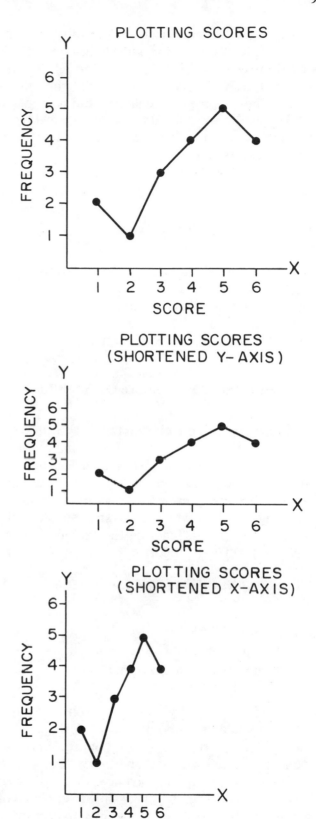

There are several ways of graphing that are numerically accurate but which may give a distorted impression of the data. Although the data are accurately plotted in each graph, the impression of the steepness of change from category to category is greatly altered by extending or shortening one of the axes. A partial corrective is the three-quarters rule.

(2) *Convention or Expectations.* If you are writing a report to a granting agency, you may want to include tables since they are usually expected.

(3) *Your Ability and Resources.* Some people are more visually astute that others and can readily place data into pleasing graphs. An electronic printer that can create tables and graphs can be helpful (although possibly expensive).

WRITING THE RESULTS OF A SURVEY

A fairly typical conclusion to a survey is a written report of its purposes, findings, and methods. One question usually immediately arises upon sitting down to organize the report: How detailed and technical should you be? If you are too technical, you might reduce your readership substantially; on the other hand, ignoring the technical details might subject your report to criticism from other surveyors.

Three aims should guide your writing.

- Be comprehensive.
- Organize carefully.
- Write as clearly as you can.

Sound like one of your earliest school teachers warning you about a book report? Perhaps. But if these three criteria are applied, your report is more likely to be read widely than otherwise.

Aiming for comprehensiveness means that you should include as much as possible to explain your survey so that anyone who wants to can understand it thoroughly. You must organize it so that anyone can find out what he or she wants to know. If I am interested in why you chose the XYZ Self-Esteem Inventory, I would like to be able to find that information fairly easily. Did you provide me with a table of contents?

Writing clearly is always a desirable aim. In survey reports, clarity means using standard English and making sure that all technical terms are defined. How might these aims be achieved?

Organizing the Report

The report should include:

- an abstract
- a summary
- a table of contents
- a list of tables and figures
- a glossary of terms
- purposes
- methods and findings
- discussion

The Abstract. Write a 150 to 250 word abstract of your survey. If you were reporting the results of a survey of community attitudes toward letting women into a traditionally all-male organization, your abstract might have this outline:

Example: The Abstract of a Survey Report

The Purpose: To find out community attitudes toward letting girls and women into the XCs—a traditionally all-male service organization.

The Methods: Telephone interviews on July 25, 1985; ten trained volunteers from the XCs.

The Sample Size and Response Rate: 150 people; 82 percent; 30 percent men.

Findings: 80 percent for; 20 percent against; 72 percent of men for; 85 percent of women for; younger people were less enthusiastic.

Cautions: Many more women in sample than men (62 percent to 38 percent); practically all nonrespondents were men.

Here is how the abstract might read:

The XCs conducted a telephone interview with 150 people on July 25, 1985, to find out community attitudes to letting women into its organization. The XCs have traditionally been male since its beginning in 1960. The sample consisted of randomly selected volunteer workers in community agencies, 82 percent of whom completed their interview. On average, 80 percent were for admission of women. Of the men, 72 percent supported admission, while 85 percent of women did. It should be noted that nearly two-thirds of the sample was female and practically all nonrespondents were men.

Summary. A summary should be included in the report. The summary is a distillation of all the report's key components (purposes, methods, findings). It can be about three pages and take about ten minutes to read. In addition to including more detail than the abstract, you should also tell who conducted the survey, what it means, and you might include one or two key tables.

For the survey of attitudes toward letting women into the XCs, you might include a table like this:

Comparison Between Men and Women on Their Answers to Two Important Questions (in percentages)

Responses	Men (N =)	Women (N =)
Agree women should be admitted		
Disagree women should be admitted		
Uncertain		
If coed, would be an active member		
wouldn't be active		
Uncertain		

Table of Contents. The table of contents should list all major sections of the report and give page numbers.

List of Tables and Figures. Each table and figure should be listed with its complete name (e.g., Figure 1: Changes in Women's Attitudes Toward Coed Business Associations from 1955 to 1985) and give the corresponding page numbers.

Glossary of Terms. All technical terms (e.g., random samples) or special abbreviations should be explained (e.g., CBS = Center for Business and Science).

Purposes. A survey's purposes are its reasons and expectations. One survey, for example, might be conducted to find out how satisfied participants are with their benefits from the XCs, while another might be performed to find out how many participants in the local XC chapter are involved in high technology and service enterprises.

Methods and Findings. These are what the surveyor did and learned. They include:

- type of survey (self-administered questionnaire, face-to-face interview) and limitations (used the telephone but would have preferred face-to-face because. . . .)
- questions asked (give examples or include the entire survey)
- survey logistics (when administered, by whom, how trained); limitations (trained five people; only four were adequate)
- survey construction (who wrote questions, pilot testing, reliability and validity statistics); limitations (reliability coefficients only .65; validity unknown)
- sampling and response rate (how selected, how adequate); limitations (hoped for response rate of 80 percent but got 70 percent, partially because one interviewer was fired and because of time, we could not make all planned follow-up calls)
- design (cross-sectional? longitudinal? comparison?); limitations (we would have preferred a panel to a cohort because. . . .)
- questions asked (sample or the entire instrument)
- findings (results of survey; if analysis method is other than numbers and percentages, specify and if necessary, explain; use tables, graphs and other visual aids)

Discussion. The discussion should connect the findings to the survey's purposes and point out any unexpected results. Consider this excerpt from a discussion section of the report of a survey to find out if community support exists for admitting girls and women into the XCs, currently an all-male business association.

Example: Discussion Section of Survey Report

The majority of men (72 percent) and women (85 percent) were for admitting girls and women into the XCs. Younger people, however, were surprisingly less unenthusiastic than some of their older counterparts. About 52 percent of the respondents that were 25 years of age or younger were definitely or probably against making the XCs coed, whereas only 32 percent of those over 25 years were. These findings may reflect the general conservative trend among young people that was evident in the community in the last election.

When you write a discussion, you must decide whether your responsibility also includes putting the data to use. Are you the one to recommend making the XCs coed? Unless you are specifically asked to plan the program or to make policy, evaluative or research decisions—the basic uses of survey data—do not do it. Here is why:

A survey is likely to be just one source for making decisions about societal welfare. Other sources include political expedience, humane and religious beliefs, and other types of empirical or judgmental data. In only rare and very specific instances, is it appropriate for the surveyor to come to conclusions alone.

Clear Writing

Some tips on clarity of items.

(1) Use the active voice whenever possible.

Poor: The report *is* relatively simple and *is* obviously written for the nonexpert for there *are* very few statistical tables given. (Twenty words; three are forms of the verb "to be.")

Better: The relatively simple report is obviously written for the nonexpert, for it *gives* very few statistical tables. (Seventeen words; 2 verbs.)

(2) Do not sprinkle sentences with prepositional phrases. When possible delete: "in order to give a reason," which can be replaced with "to give a reason." Convert a prepositional phrase to a participle: "In the effort to get reliable attitude measures" can become "Trying to get re-liable attitude measures." Convert a prepositional phrase to an adjective: "It is a question of importance" can become "It is an important question"

Replace	With
at an early date	soon
at the present time	now
in order to	to
prior to	before
subsequent to	after

(3) Try a readability formula. Readability testing predicts the grade level of written material. At least one expert has said that the Gettysburg Address, *Time,* and *Newsweek* are written at the tenth-grade level. Most people feel comfortable reading below their level. Here is how to complete one readability index, the FOG Index.

(1) Take a 100-word sample of your survey report.
(2) Compute the average number of words per sentence. If the final sentence in your sample runs beyond 100 words, use the total number of words at the end of that sentence to compute the average.
(3) Count the number of words in the 100-word sample with more than two syllables. Do not count proper nouns or three-syllable word forms ending in -ed or -es.
(4) Add the average number of words per sentence to the number of words containing more than two syllables and multiply the sum by 0.4.

Example: Suppose a 100-word passage contains an average of 20 words per sentence and ten words of more than two syllables. The sum of these is 30. Multiplying 30 by 0.4 gives a FOG Index of the twelfth grade.

THE ORAL PRESENTATION

Oral presentations follow many of the rules of written reports. Speak clearly and slowly and pace your presentation to the audience's needs.

One important difference is that because oral presentations are timed, you cannot always give a comprehensive account of the survey. You must be selective, an often difficult task. Among the criteria for selecting topics to talk about is the relative importance of the different aspects of the survey. Usually people are primarily concerned with who participated and what was found. If you have time, you can talk about the survey's methods and limits.

Another criterion for selecting topics to report depends upon how meaningful the data will be. If you have fully completed one portion of the survey and are ready to analyze and review the accuracy of data collected on some other, only tell about the completed portion.

To help your presentation, always consider using handouts or visual aids like slides and transparancies. (If they are available and relevant, visual aids like films and videotapes can sometimes enliven a presentation.)

Handouts. These usually consist of tables describing the respondents' or the survey's findings. Make sure that your tables are readable, but do not assume anyone will read them. To make sure everyone does, draw attention to the tables and then go through each one step by step. Explain the title, all headings, the source of data, and what the numbers mean (averages? percentages?).

Transparencies. Limit each transparency to one topic or concept. Keep it as simple as possible by limiting copy to six lines per transparency and six words per line. The type should be at least eighteen point (one-quarter-inch high). Do not use a pica or elite typewriter, only a primary size. Avoid running your text closer than three-eighths inch from the edges after allowing room for mounting. Again, choose active verbs and short sentences when you are presenting verbal material, and make the tables and graphs as easy to read as possible. Do not forget to go over all tables and all graphs with the audience. Make sure they understand the titles, the source of information, and what the numbers mean. Be careful of using copyrighted material. You cannot automatically assume that you have permission to use anything from a newspaper, journal, or magazine. It is extremely important to make sure that before you begin your presentation, your transparencies are in the correct order and proper side up.

Slides. One of the most effective methods of reporting data is to show them on a slide. The real art of preparing slides is what you select to be on them. The first rule: Be as simple as you can. Do not clutter the slide with too many lines, bars, or numbers. Remember, for every slide, people listening to your report must do several things simultaneously: listen to you, read the slide, and interpret its meaning.

What goes into a slide, and how should it be prepared? Very few people photograph their own slides; professionals exist that can be found in almost any good camera store who can tell you the requirements for a visually satisfying slide of your data. They will tell you if the slide should be blue with white numbers and letters (effective for tables and easy on the eyes) or if you should use other colors to set off a pie diagram, for example.

Here are some guidelines for preparing slides.

(1) Use graph paper to discipline yourself to stay within boundaries: about fifty spaces across and about seventeen down.

(2) If you have a table that does not occupy all available spaces, place it in the center rather than at the edges:

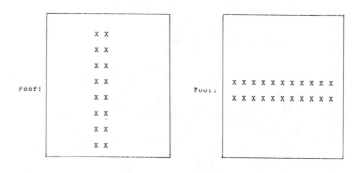

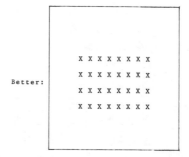

(3) Use full capitals or oversize or larger than ordinary type. For example:

WHO COMES TO THE CENTER?

- ALMOST ALL WERE BETWEEN 20 AND 21

- 77 WERE FROM MINORITY BACK-GROUNDS

- ALMOST 40 PERCENT LIVED WITH JUST THEIR MOTHER

- OVER 75 PERCENT WERE IN SCHOOL

(4) Present the summary data (such as percentages or means). Look at this slide used in a report of an interview conducted in July 1984, with the medical directors of sixteen clinics, fifteen of which were in an experimental program and one of which served as a control. Compare it with the data from which it was taken.

Example: Data Used to Make a Slide

Average Number and Range of Days a Patient with an Acute Problem Must Wait to See His/Her Regular Provider or Any Provider

	Waiting Time in Days Assuming the Provider Is Specifically Named and Is			Waiting Time for	
Site	Medical Director or Faculty	House Staff	Nurse Practitioner (NP) or Physician Assistant (PA)	Any Practice Physician	Any Practice Provider
F	1.6	11.5	2.5	NA	NA
G	.8	13.0(1)	NA	0.0	0.0
A	1.9	0.0	0.0	0.0	NA
J	.7	1.5	0.0	0.0	0.0
B	2.7	.7	1.8	.2	.2
L	16.8(1)	3.7	NA	0.0	NA
I	1.2	1.2	1.0	0.0	0.0
N	3.8	15.0(3)	9.8	0.0	0.0
C	.8	.2	0.0	0.0	0.0
O	0.0	3.1	NA	0.0	NA
D	16.7	15.7(1)	1.2	1.0	.6
P	11.8(1)	2.4	0.0	0.0	0.0
E	13.4	20.6(3)	.5	.3	.3
H	.5	2.3	.2	0.0	.2
K	1.3	1.3	NA	0.0	0.0
All Sites	4.9	6.1	1.5	.1	.1
Control	24.8(2)	8.7	1.5	NA	NA

NOTE: Numbers in parentheses represent the number of providers for whom patients must wait more than 30 days to schedule an appointment. For example, at site G, one of the house staff named was not available for at least 30 days. NA = not applicable or no data available.

Example: Slide from Data in Table N

NUMBER OF DAYS AN ESTABLISHED PATIENT WITH AN ACUTE PROBLEM MUST WAIT TO SEE REGULAR PROVIDER OR ANY PROVIDER

REGULAR PROVIDER	EXPERIMENTAL SITES	CONTROL GROUP
	MEAN (RANGE)	MEAN
FACULTY M.D.	4.9 (0.0-16.8)	24.8
HOUSE STAFF	6.1 (0.0-20.6)	8.7
NP/PA	1.5 (1.0-9.8)	1.5
ANY PRACTICE PHYSICIAN	0.1 (0.0-1.0)	NA
ANY PRACTICE PROVIDER	0.1 (0.0-0.6)	NA

APPENDIX

TABLE A1
Random Numbers

03 47 43 73 86	36 96 47 36 61	46 98 63 71 62	33 26 16 80 45	60 11 14 10 95
97 74 24 67 62	42 81 14 57 20	42 53 32 37 32	27 07 36 07 51	24 51 79 89 73
16 76 62 27 66	56 50 26 71 07	32 90 79 78 53	13 55 38 58 59	88 97 54 14 10
12 56 85 99 26	96 96 68 27 31	05 03 72 93 15	57 12 10 14 21	88 26 49 81 76
55 59 56 35 64	38 54 82 46 22	31 62 43 09 90	06 18 44 32 53	23 83 01 30 30
16 22 77 94 39	49 54 43 54 82	17 37 93 23 78	87 35 20 96 43	84 26 34 91 64
84 42 17 53 31	57 24 55 06 88	77 04 74 47 67	21 76 33 50 25	83 92 12 06 76
63 01 63 78 59	16 95 55 67 19	98 10 50 71 75	12 86 73 58 07	44 39 52 38 79
33 21 12 34 29	78 64 56 07 82	52 42 07 44 38	15 51 00 13 42	99 66 02 79 54
57 60 86 32 44	09 47 27 96 54	49 17 46 09 62	90 52 84 77 27	08 02 73 43 28
18 18 07 92 46	44 17 16 58 09	79 83 86 19 62	06 76 50 03 10	55 23 64 05 05
26 62 38 97 75	84 16 07 44 99	83 11 46 32 24	20 14 85 88 45	10 93 72 88 71
23 42 40 64 74	82 97 77 77 81	07 45 32 14 08	32 98 94 07 72	93 85 79 10 75
52 36 28 19 95	50 92 26 11 97	00 56 76 31 38	80 22 02 53 53	86 60 42 04 53
37 85 94 35 12	83 39 50 08 30	42 34 07 96 88	54 42 06 87 98	35 85 29 48 39
70 29 17 12 13	40 33 20 38 26	13 89 51 03 74	17 76 37 13 04	07 74 21 19 30
56 62 18 37 35	96 83 50 87 75	97 12 25 93 47	70 33 24 03 54	97 77 46 44 80
99 49 57 22 77	88 42 95 45 72	16 64 36 16 00	04 43 18 66 79	94 77 24 21 90
16 08 15 04 72	33 27 14 34 09	45 59 34 68 49	12 72 07 34 45	99 27 72 95 14
31 16 93 32 43	50 27 89 87 19	20 15 37 00 49	52 85 66 60 44	38 68 88 11 80
68 34 30 13 70	55 74 30 77 40	44 22 78 84 26	04 33 46 09 52	68 07 97 06 57
74 57 25 65 76	59 29 97 68 60	71 91 38 67 54	13 58 18 24 76	15 54 55 95 52
27 42 37 86 53	48 55 90 65 72	96 57 69 36 10	96 46 92 42 45	97 60 49 04 91
00 39 68 29 61	66 37 32 20 30	77 84 57 03 29	10 45 65 04 26	11 04 96 67 24
29 94 98 94 24	68 49 69 10 82	53 75 91 93 30	34 25 20 57 27	40 48 73 51 92
16 90 82 66 59	83 62 64 11 12	67 19 00 71 74	60 47 21 29 68	02 02 37 03 31
11 27 94 75 06	06 09 19 74 66	02 94 37 34 02	76 70 90 30 86	38 45 94 30 38
35 24 10 16 20	33 32 51 26 38	79 78 45 04 91	16 92 53 56 16	02 75 50 95 98
38 23 16 86 38	42 38 97 01 50	87 75 66 81 41	40 01 74 91 62	48 51 84 08 32
31 96 25 91 47	96 44 33 49 13	34 86 82 53 91	00 52 43 48 85	27 55 26 89 62
56 67 40 67 14	64 05 71 95 86	11 05 65 09 68	76 83 20 37 90	57 16 00 11 66
14 90 84 45 11	75 73 88 05 90	52 27 41 14 86	22 98 12 22 08	07 52 74 95 80
68 05 51 18 00	33 96 02 75 19	07 60 62 93 55	59 33 82 43 90	49 37 38 44,59
20 46 78 73 90	97 51 40 14 02	04 02 33 31 08	39 54 16 49 36	47 95 93 13 30
64 19 58 97 79	15 06 15 93 20	01 90 10 75 06	40 78 78 89 62	02 67 74 17 33
05 26 93 70 60	22 35 85 15 13	92 03 51 59 77	59 56 78 06 83	52 91 05 70 74
07 97 10 88 23	09 98 42 99 64	61 71 62 99 15	06 51 29 16 93	58 05 77 09 51
68 71 86 85 85	54 87 66 47 54	73 32 08 11 12	44 95 92 63 16	29 56 24 29 48
26 99 61 65 53	58 37 78 80 70	42 10 50 67 42	32 17 55 85 74	94 44 67 16 94
14 65 52 68 75	87 59 36 22 41	26 78 63 06 55	13 08 27 01 50	15 29 39 39 43
17 53 77 58 71	71 41 61 50 72	12 41 94 96 26	44 95 27 36 99	02 96 74 30 83
90 26 59 21 19	23 52 23 33 12	96 93 02 18 39	07 02 18 36 07	25 99 32 70 23
41 23 52 55 99	31 04 49 69 96	10 47 48 45 88	13 41 43 89 20	97 17 14 49 17
60 20 50 81 69	31 99 73 68 68	35 81 33 03 76	24 30 12 48 60	18 99 10 72 34
91 25 38 05 90	94 58 28 41 36	45 37 59 03 09	90 35 57 29 12	82 62 54 65 60
34 50 57 74 37	98 80 33 00 91	09 77 93 19 82	74 94 80 04 04	45 07 31 66 49
85 22 04 39 43	73 81 53 94 79	33 62 46 86 28	08 31 54 46 31	53 94 13 38 47
09 79 13 77 48	73 82 97 22 21	05 03 27 24 83	72 89 44 05 60	35 80 39 94 88
88 75 80 18 14	22 95 75 42 49	39 32 82 22 49	02 48 07 70 37	16 04 61 67 87
90 96 23 70 00	39 00 03 06 90	55 85 78 38 36	94 37 30 69 32	90 89 00 76 33

SOURCE: This table is taken from Table XXXIII in Fisher and Yates: *Statistical Tables for Biological, Agricultural and Medical Research*, Published by Longman Group, Ltd. London (previously published by Oliver & Boyd Ltd. Edinburgh) and by permission of the authors and publishers.

TABLE A2
Distribution of F

$n_2{}^a$	\multicolumn{24}{c}{n_1 degrees of freedom (for greater mean square)}

$n_2{}^a$	1	2	3	4	5	6	7	8	9	10	11	12	14	16	20	24	30	40	50	75	100	200	500	∞
1	161	200	216	225	230	234	237	239	241	242	243	244	245	246	248	249	250	251	252	253	253	254	254	254
	4,052	4,999	5,403	5,625	5,764	5,859	5,928	5,981	6,022	6,056	6,082	6,106	6,142	6,169	6,208	6,234	6,258	6,286	6,302	6,323	6,334	6,352	6,361	6,366
2	18.51	19.00	19.16	19.25	19.30	19.33	19.36	19.37	19.38	19.39	19.40	19.41	19.42	19.43	19.44	19.45	19.46	19.47	19.47	19.48	19.49	19.49	19.50	19.50
	98.49	99.00	99.17	99.25	99.30	99.33	99.34	99.36	99.38	99.40	99.41	99.42	99.43	99.44	99.45	99.46	99.47	99.48	99.48	99.49	99.49	99.49	99.50	99.50
3	10.13	9.55	9.28	9.12	9.01	8.94	8.88	8.84	8.81	8.78	8.76	8.74	8.71	8.69	8.66	8.64	8.62	8.60	8.58	8.57	8.56	8.54	8.54	8.53
	34.12	30.82	29.46	28.71	28.24	27.91	27.67	27.49	27.34	27.23	27.13	27.05	26.92	26.83	26.69	26.60	26.50	26.41	26.35	26.27	26.23	26.18	26.14	26.12
4	7.71	6.94	6.59	6.39	6.26	6.16	6.09	6.04	6.00	5.96	5.93	5.91	5.87	5.84	5.80	5.77	5.74	5.71	5.70	5.68	5.66	5.65	5.64	5.63
	21.20	18.00	16.69	15.98	15.52	15.21	14.98	14.80	14.66	14.54	14.45	14.37	14.24	14.15	14.02	13.93	13.83	13.74	13.69	13.61	13.57	13.52	13.48	13.46
5	6.61	5.79	5.41	5.19	5.05	4.95	4.88	4.82	4.78	4.74	4.70	4.68	4.64	4.60	4.56	4.53	4.50	4.46	4.44	4.42	4.40	4.38	4.37	4.36
	16.26	13.27	12.06	11.39	10.97	10.67	10.45	10.27	10.15	10.05	9.96	9.89	9.77	9.68	9.55	9.47	9.38	9.29	9.24	9.17	9.13	9.07	9.04	9.02
6	5.99	5.14	4.76	4.53	4.39	4.28	4.21	4.15	4.10	4.06	4.03	4.00	3.96	3.92	3.87	3.84	3.81	3.77	3.75	3.72	3.71	3.69	3.68	3.67
	13.74	10.92	9.78	9.15	8.75	8.47	8.26	8.10	7.98	7.87	7.79	7.72	7.60	7.52	7.39	7.31	7.23	7.14	7.09	7.02	6.99	6.94	6.90	6.88
7	5.59	4.74	4.35	4.12	3.97	3.87	3.79	3.73	3.68	3.63	3.60	3.57	3.52	3.49	3.44	3.41	3.38	3.34	3.32	3.29	3.28	3.25	3.24	3.23
	12.25	9.55	8.45	7.85	7.46	7.19	7.00	6.84	6.71	6.62	6.54	6.47	6.35	6.27	6.15	6.07	5.98	5.90	5.85	5.78	5.75	5.70	5.67	5.65
8	5.32	4.46	4.07	3.84	3.69	3.58	3.50	3.44	3.39	3.34	3.31	3.28	3.23	3.20	3.15	3.12	3.08	3.05	3.03	3.00	2.98	2.96	2.94	2.93
	11.26	8.65	7.59	7.01	6.63	6.37	6.19	6.03	5.91	5.82	5.74	5.67	5.56	5.48	5.36	5.28	5.20	5.11	5.06	5.00	4.96	4.91	4.88	4.86
9	5.12	4.26	3.86	3.63	3.48	3.37	3.29	3.23	3.18	3.13	3.10	3.07	3.02	2.98	2.93	2.90	2.86	2.82	2.80	2.77	2.76	2.73	2.72	2.71
	10.56	8.02	6.99	6.42	6.06	5.80	5.62	5.47	5.35	5.26	5.18	5.11	5.00	4.92	4.80	4.73	4.64	4.56	4.51	4.45	4.41	4.36	4.33	4.31
10	4.96	4.10	3.71	3.48	3.33	3.22	3.14	3.07	3.02	2.97	2.94	2.91	2.86	2.82	2.77	2.74	2.70	2.67	2.64	2.61	2.59	2.56	2.55	2.54
	10.04	7.56	6.55	5.99	5.64	5.39	5.21	5.06	4.95	4.85	4.78	4.71	4.60	4.52	4.41	4.33	4.25	4.17	4.12	4.05	4.01	3.96	3.93	3.91
11	4.84	3.98	3.59	3.36	3.20	3.09	3.01	2.95	2.90	2.86	2.82	2.79	2.74	2.70	2.65	2.61	2.57	2.53	2.50	2.47	2.45	2.42	2.41	2.40
	9.65	7.20	6.22	5.67	5.32	5.07	4.88	4.74	4.63	4.54	4.46	4.40	4.29	4.21	4.10	4.02	3.94	3.86	3.80	3.74	3.70	3.66	3.62	3.60
12	4.75	3.88	3.49	3.26	3.11	3.00	2.92	2.85	2.80	2.76	2.72	2.69	2.64	2.60	2.54	2.50	2.46	2.42	2.40	2.36	2.35	2.32	2.31	2.30
	9.33	6.93	5.95	5.41	5.06	4.82	4.65	4.50	4.39	4.30	4.22	4.16	4.05	3.98	3.86	3.78	3.70	3.61	3.56	3.49	3.46	3.41	3.38	3.36
13	4.67	3.80	3.41	3.18	3.02	2.92	2.84	2.77	2.72	2.67	2.63	2.60	2.55	2.51	2.46	2.42	2.38	2.34	2.32	2.28	2.26	2.24	2.22	2.21
	9.07	6.70	5.74	5.20	4.86	4.62	4.44	4.30	4.19	4.10	4.02	3.96	3.85	3.78	3.67	3.59	3.51	3.42	3.37	3.30	3.27	3.21	3.18	3.16
14	4.60	3.74	3.34	3.11	2.96	2.85	2.77	2.70	2.65	2.60	2.56	2.53	2.48	2.44	2.39	2.35	2.31	2.27	2.24	2.21	2.19	2.16	2.14	2.13
	8.86	6.51	5.56	5.03	4.69	4.46	4.28	4.14	4.03	3.94	3.86	3.80	3.70	3.62	3.51	3.43	3.34	3.26	3.21	3.14	3.11	3.06	3.02	3.00
15	4.54	3.68	3.29	3.06	2.90	2.79	2.70	2.64	2.59	2.55	2.51	2.48	2.43	2.39	2.33	2.29	2.25	2.21	2.18	2.15	2.12	2.10	2.08	2.07
	8.68	6.36	5.42	4.89	4.56	4.32	4.14	4.00	3.89	3.80	3.73	3.67	3.56	3.48	3.36	3.29	3.20	3.12	3.07	3.00	2.97	2.92	2.89	2.87
16	4.49	3.63	3.24	3.01	2.85	2.74	2.66	2.59	2.54	2.49	2.45	2.42	2.37	2.33	2.28	2.24	2.20	2.16	2.13	2.09	2.07	2.04	2.02	2.01
	8.53	6.23	5.29	4.77	4.44	4.20	4.03	3.89	3.78	3.69	3.61	3.55	3.45	3.37	3.25	3.18	3.10	3.01	2.96	2.89	2.86	2.80	2.77	2.75
17	4.45	3.59	3.20	2.96	2.81	2.70	2.62	2.55	2.50	2.45	2.41	2.38	2.33	2.29	2.23	2.19	2.15	2.11	2.08	2.04	2.02	1.99	1.97	1.96
	8.40	6.11	5.18	4.67	4.34	4.10	3.93	3.79	3.68	3.59	3.52	3.45	3.35	3.27	3.16	3.08	3.00	2.92	2.86	2.79	2.76	2.70	2.67	2.65
18	4.41	3.55	3.16	2.93	2.77	2.66	2.58	2.51	2.46	2.41	2.37	2.34	2.29	2.25	2.19	2.15	2.11	2.07	2.04	2.00	1.98	1.95	1.93	1.92
	8.28	6.01	5.09	4.58	4.25	4.01	3.85	3.71	3.60	3.51	3.44	3.37	3.27	3.19	3.07	3.00	2.91	2.83	2.78	2.71	2.68	2.62	2.59	2.57
19	4.38	3.52	3.13	2.90	2.74	2.63	2.55	2.48	2.43	2.38	2.34	2.31	2.26	2.21	2.15	2.11	2.07	2.02	2.00	1.96	1.94	1.91	1.90	1.88
	8.18	5.93	5.01	4.50	4.17	3.94	3.77	3.63	3.52	3.43	3.36	3.30	3.19	3.12	3.00	2.92	2.84	2.76	2.70	2.63	2.60	2.54	2.51	2.49
20	4.35	3.49	3.10	2.87	2.71	2.60	2.52	2.45	2.40	2.35	2.31	2.28	2.23	2.18	2.12	2.08	2.04	1.99	1.96	1.92	1.90	1.87	1.85	1.84
	8.10	5.85	4.94	4.43	4.10	3.87	3.71	3.56	3.45	3.37	3.30	3.23	3.13	3.05	2.94	2.86	2.77	2.69	2.63	2.56	2.53	2.47	2.44	2.42
21	4.32	3.47	3.07	2.84	2.68	2.57	2.49	2.42	2.37	2.32	2.28	2.25	2.20	2.15	2.09	2.05	2.00	1.96	1.93	1.89	1.87	1.84	1.82	1.81
	8.02	5.78	4.87	4.37	4.04	3.81	3.65	3.51	3.40	3.31	3.24	3.17	3.07	2.99	2.88	2.80	2.72	2.63	2.58	2.51	2.47	2.42	2.38	2.36
22	4.30	3.44	3.05	2.82	2.66	2.55	2.47	2.40	2.35	2.30	2.26	2.23	2.18	2.13	2.07	2.03	1.98	1.93	1.91	1.87	1.84	1.81	1.80	1.78
	7.94	5.72	4.82	4.31	3.99	3.76	3.59	3.45	3.35	3.26	3.18	3.12	3.02	2.94	2.83	2.75	2.67	2.58	2.53	2.46	2.42	2.37	2.33	2.31
23	4.28	3.42	3.03	2.80	2.64	2.53	2.45	2.38	2.32	2.28	2.24	2.20	2.14	2.10	2.04	2.00	1.96	1.91	1.88	1.84	1.82	1.79	1.77	1.76
	7.88	5.66	4.76	4.26	3.94	3.71	3.54	3.41	3.30	3.21	3.14	3.07	2.97	2.89	2.78	2.70	2.62	2.53	2.48	2.41	2.37	2.32	2.28	2.26
24	4.26	3.40	3.01	2.78	2.62	2.51	2.43	2.36	2.30	2.26	2.22	2.18	2.13	2.09	2.02	1.98	1.94	1.89	1.86	1.82	1.80	1.76	1.74	1.73
	7.82	5.61	4.72	4.22	3.90	3.67	3.50	3.36	3.25	3.17	3.09	3.03	2.93	2.85	2.74	2.66	2.58	2.49	2.44	2.36	2.33	2.27	2.23	2.21
25	4.24	3.38	2.99	2.76	2.60	2.49	2.41	2.34	2.28	2.24	2.20	2.16	2.11	2.06	2.00	1.96	1.92	1.87	1.84	1.80	1.77	1.74	1.72	1.71
	7.77	5.57	4.68	4.18	3.86	3.63	3.46	3.32	3.21	3.13	3.05	2.99	2.89	2.81	2.70	2.62	2.54	2.45	2.40	2.32	2.29	2.23	2.19	2.17
26	4.22	3.37	2.98	2.74	2.59	2.47	2.39	2.32	2.27	2.22	2.18	2.15	2.10	2.05	1.99	1.95	1.90	1.85	1.82	1.78	1.76	1.72	1.70	1.69
	7.72	5.53	4.64	4.14	3.82	3.59	3.42	3.29	3.17	3.09	3.02	2.96	2.86	2.77	2.66	2.58	2.50	2.41	2.36	2.28	2.25	2.19	2.15	2.13

TABLE A2 Continued

n_2[a]	\multicolumn{24}{c}{n_1 degrees of freedom (for greater mean square)}

n_2	1	2	3	4	5	6	7	8	9	10	11	12	14	16	20	24	30	40	50	75	100	200	500	∞
27	4.21	3.35	2.96	2.73	2.57	2.46	2.37	2.30	2.25	2.20	2.16	2.13	2.08	2.03	1.97	1.93	1.88	1.84	1.80	1.76	1.74	1.71	1.68	1.67
	7.68	5.49	4.60	4.11	3.79	3.56	3.39	3.26	3.14	3.06	2.98	2.93	2.83	2.74	2.63	2.55	2.47	2.38	2.33	2.25	2.21	2.16	2.12	2.10
28	4.20	3.34	2.95	2.71	2.56	2.44	2.36	2.29	2.24	2.19	2.15	2.12	2.06	2.02	1.96	1.91	1.87	1.81	1.78	1.75	1.72	1.69	1.67	1.65
	7.64	5.45	4.57	4.07	3.76	3.53	3.36	3.23	3.11	3.03	2.95	2.90	2.80	2.71	2.60	2.52	2.44	2.35	2.30	2.22	2.18	2.13	2.09	2.06
29	4.18	3.33	2.93	2.70	2.54	2.43	2.35	2.28	2.22	2.18	2.14	2.10	2.05	2.00	1.94	1.90	1.85	1.80	1.77	1.73	1.71	1.68	1.65	1.64
	7.60	5.42	4.54	4.04	3.73	3.50	3.33	3.20	3.08	3.00	2.92	2.87	2.77	2.68	2.57	2.49	2.41	2.32	2.27	2.19	2.15	2.10	2.06	2.03
30	4.17	3.32	2.92	2.69	2.53	2.42	2.34	2.27	2.21	2.16	2.12	2.09	2.04	1.99	1.93	1.89	1.84	1.79	1.76	1.72	1.69	1.66	1.64	1.62
	7.56	5.39	4.51	4.02	3.70	3.47	3.30	3.17	3.06	2.98	2.90	2.84	2.74	2.66	2.55	2.47	2.38	2.29	2.24	2.16	2.13	2.07	2.03	2.01
32	4.15	3.30	2.90	2.67	2.51	2.40	2.32	2.25	2.19	2.14	2.10	2.07	2.02	1.97	1.91	1.86	1.82	1.76	1.74	1.69	1.67	1.64	1.61	1.59
	7.50	5.34	4.46	3.97	3.66	3.42	3.25	3.12	3.01	2.94	2.86	2.80	2.70	2.62	2.51	2.42	2.34	2.25	2.20	2.12	2.08	2.02	1.98	1.96
34	4.13	3.28	2.88	2.65	2.49	2.38	2.30	2.23	2.17	2.12	2.08	2.05	2.00	1.95	1.89	1.84	1.80	1.74	1.71	1.67	1.64	1.61	1.59	1.57
	7.44	5.29	4.42	3.93	3.61	3.38	3.21	3.08	2.97	2.89	2.82	2.76	2.66	2.58	2.47	2.38	2.30	2.21	2.15	2.08	2.04	1.98	1.94	1.91
36	4.11	3.26	2.86	2.63	2.48	2.36	2.28	2.21	2.15	2.10	2.06	2.03	1.98	1.93	1.87	1.82	1.78	1.72	1.69	1.65	1.62	1.59	1.56	1.55
	7.39	5.25	4.38	3.89	3.58	3.35	3.18	3.04	2.94	2.86	2.78	2.72	2.62	2.54	2.43	2.35	2.26	2.17	2.12	2.04	2.00	1.94	1.90	1.87
38	4.10	3.25	2.85	2.62	2.46	2.35	2.26	2.19	2.14	2.09	2.05	2.02	1.96	1.92	1.85	1.80	1.76	1.71	1.67	1.63	1.60	1.57	1.54	1.53
	7.35	5.21	4.34	3.86	3.54	3.32	3.15	3.02	2.91	2.82	2.75	2.69	2.59	2.51	2.40	2.32	2.22	2.14	2.08	2.00	1.97	1.90	1.86	1.84
40	4.08	3.23	2.84	2.61	2.45	2.34	2.25	2.18	2.12	2.07	2.04	2.00	1.95	1.90	1.84	1.79	1.74	1.69	1.66	1.61	1.59	1.55	1.53	1.51
	7.31	5.18	4.31	3.83	3.51	3.29	3.12	2.99	2.88	2.80	2.73	2.66	2.56	2.49	2.37	2.29	2.20	2.11	2.05	1.97	1.94	1.88	1.84	1.81
42	4.07	3.22	2.83	2.59	2.44	2.32	2.24	2.17	2.11	2.06	2.02	1.99	1.94	1.89	1.82	1.78	1.73	1.68	1.64	1.60	1.57	1.54	1.51	1.49
	7.27	5.15	4.29	3.80	3.49	3.26	3.10	2.96	2.86	2.77	2.70	2.64	2.54	2.46	2.35	2.26	2.17	2.08	2.02	1.94	1.91	1.85	1.80	1.78
44	4.06	3.21	2.82	2.58	2.43	2.31	2.23	2.16	2.10	2.05	2.01	1.98	1.92	1.88	1.81	1.76	1.72	1.66	1.63	1.58	1.56	1.52	1.50	1.48
	7.24	5.12	4.26	3.78	3.46	3.24	3.07	2.94	2.84	2.75	2.68	2.62	2.52	2.44	2.32	2.24	2.15	2.06	2.00	1.92	1.88	1.82	1.78	1.75
46	4.05	3.20	2.81	2.57	2.42	2.30	2.22	2.14	2.09	2.04	2.00	1.97	1.91	1.87	1.80	1.75	1.71	1.65	1.62	1.57	1.54	1.51	1.48	1.46
	7.21	5.10	4.24	3.76	3.44	3.22	3.05	2.92	2.82	2.73	2.66	2.60	2.50	2.42	2.30	2.22	2.13	2.04	1.98	1.90	1.86	1.80	1.76	1.72
48	4.04	3.19	2.80	2.56	2.41	2.30	2.21	2.14	2.08	2.03	1.99	1.96	1.90	1.86	1.79	1.74	1.70	1.64	1.61	1.56	1.53	1.50	1.47	1.45
	7.19	5.08	4.22	3.74	3.42	3.20	3.04	2.90	2.80	2.71	2.64	2.58	2.48	2.40	2.28	2.20	2.11	2.02	1.96	1.88	1.84	1.78	1.73	1.70
50	4.03	3.18	2.79	2.56	2.40	2.29	2.20	2.13	2.07	2.02	1.98	1.95	1.90	1.85	1.78	1.74	1.69	1.63	1.60	1.55	1.52	1.48	1.46	1.44
	7.17	5.06	4.20	3.72	3.41	3.18	3.02	2.88	2.78	2.70	2.62	2.56	2.46	2.39	2.26	2.18	2.10	2.00	1.94	1.86	1.82	1.76	1.71	1.68
55	4.02	3.17	2.78	2.54	2.38	2.27	2.18	2.11	2.05	2.00	1.97	1.93	1.88	1.83	1.76	1.72	1.67	1.61	1.58	1.52	1.50	1.46	1.43	1.41
	7.12	5.01	4.16	3.68	3.37	3.15	2.98	2.85	2.75	2.66	2.59	2.53	2.43	2.35	2.23	2.15	2.06	1.96	1.90	1.82	1.78	1.71	1.66	1.64
60	4.00	3.15	2.76	2.52	2.37	2.25	2.17	2.10	2.04	1.99	1.95	1.92	1.86	1.81	1.75	1.70	1.65	1.59	1.56	1.50	1.48	1.44	1.41	1.39
	7.08	4.98	4.13	3.65	3.34	3.12	2.95	2.82	2.72	2.63	2.56	2.50	2.40	2.32	2.20	2.12	2.03	1.93	1.87	1.79	1.74	1.68	1.63	1.60
65	3.99	3.14	2.75	2.51	2.36	2.24	2.15	2.08	2.02	1.98	1.94	1.90	1.85	1.80	1.73	1.68	1.63	1.57	1.54	1.49	1.46	1.42	1.39	1.37
	7.04	4.95	4.10	3.62	3.31	3.09	2.93	2.79	2.70	2.61	2.54	2.47	2.37	2.30	2.18	2.09	2.00	1.90	1.84	1.76	1.71	1.64	1.60	1.56
70	3.98	3.13	2.74	2.50	2.35	2.23	2.14	2.07	2.01	1.97	1.93	1.89	1.84	1.79	1.72	1.67	1.62	1.56	1.53	1.47	1.45	1.40	1.37	1.35
	7.01	4.92	4.08	3.60	3.29	3.07	2.91	2.77	2.67	2.59	2.51	2.45	2.35	2.28	2.15	2.07	1.98	1.88	1.82	1.74	1.69	1.62	1.56	1.53
80	3.96	3.11	2.72	2.48	2.33	2.21	2.12	2.05	1.99	1.95	1.91	1.88	1.82	1.77	1.70	1.65	1.60	1.54	1.51	1.45	1.42	1.38	1.35	1.32
	6.96	4.88	4.04	3.56	3.25	3.04	2.87	2.74	2.64	2.55	2.48	2.41	2.32	2.24	2.11	2.03	1.94	1.84	1.78	1.70	1.65	1.57	1.52	1.49
100	3.94	3.09	2.70	2.46	2.30	2.19	2.10	2.03	1.97	1.92	1.88	1.85	1.79	1.75	1.68	1.63	1.57	1.51	1.48	1.42	1.39	1.34	1.30	1.28
	6.90	4.82	3.98	3.51	3.20	2.99	2.82	2.69	2.59	2.51	2.43	2.36	2.26	2.19	2.06	1.98	1.89	1.79	1.73	1.64	1.59	1.51	1.46	1.43
125	3.92	3.07	2.68	2.44	2.29	2.17	2.08	2.01	1.95	1.90	1.86	1.83	1.77	1.72	1.65	1.60	1.55	1.49	1.45	1.39	1.36	1.31	1.27	1.25
	6.84	4.78	3.94	3.47	3.17	2.95	2.79	2.65	2.56	2.47	2.40	2.33	2.23	2.15	2.03	1.94	1.85	1.75	1.68	1.59	1.54	1.46	1.40	1.37
150	3.91	3.06	2.67	2.43	2.27	2.16	2.07	2.00	1.94	1.89	1.85	1.82	1.76	1.71	1.64	1.59	1.54	1.47	1.44	1.37	1.34	1.29	1.25	1.22
	6.81	4.75	3.91	3.44	3.14	2.92	2.76	2.62	2.53	2.44	2.37	2.30	2.20	2.12	2.00	1.91	1.83	1.72	1.66	1.56	1.51	1.43	1.37	1.33
200	3.89	3.04	2.65	2.41	2.26	2.14	2.05	1.98	1.92	1.87	1.83	1.80	1.74	1.69	1.62	1.57	1.52	1.45	1.42	1.35	1.32	1.26	1.22	1.19
	6.76	4.71	3.88	3.41	3.11	2.90	2.73	2.60	2.50	2.41	2.34	2.28	2.17	2.09	1.97	1.88	1.79	1.69	1.62	1.53	1.48	1.39	1.33	1.28
400	3.86	3.02	2.62	2.39	2.23	2.12	2.03	1.96	1.90	1.85	1.81	1.78	1.72	1.67	1.60	1.54	1.49	1.42	1.38	1.32	1.28	1.22	1.16	1.13
	6.70	4.66	3.83	3.36	3.06	2.85	2.69	2.55	2.46	2.37	2.29	2.23	2.12	2.04	1.92	1.84	1.74	1.64	1.57	1.47	1.42	1.32	1.24	1.19
1000	3.85	3.00	2.61	2.38	2.22	2.10	2.02	1.95	1.89	1.84	1.80	1.76	1.70	1.65	1.58	1.53	1.47	1.41	1.36	1.30	1.26	1.19	1.13	1.08
	6.66	4.62	3.80	3.34	3.04	2.82	2.66	2.53	2.43	2.34	2.26	2.20	2.09	2.01	1.89	1.81	1.71	1.61	1.54	1.44	1.38	1.28	1.19	1.11
∞	3.84	2.99	2.60	2.37	2.21	2.09	2.01	1.94	1.88	1.83	1.79	1.75	1.69	1.64	1.57	1.52	1.46	1.40	1.35	1.28	1.24	1.17	1.11	1.00
	6.64	4.60	3.78	3.32	3.02	2.80	2.64	2.51	2.41	2.32	2.24	2.18	2.07	1.99	1.87	1.79	1.69	1.59	1.52	1.41	1.36	1.25	1.15	1.00

SOURCE: Reprinted by permission from *Statistical Methods* by George W. Snedecor and William G. Cochran © 1980 by the Ohio State University Press, Ames, Iowa 50010.
NOTE: The function, $F = e$ with exponent $2z$, is computed in part from Fisher's table VI(7). Additional entries are by interpolation, mostly graphical.

a. n_2 = degrees of freedom for the lesser mean squared.

TABLE A3
Distribution of t

Probability.

n^a	.9	.8	.7	.6	.5	.4	.3	.2	.1	.05	.02	.01	.001
1	·158	·325	·510	·727	1·000	1·376	1·963	3·078	6·314	12·706	31·821	63·657	636·619
2	·142	·289	·445	·617	·816	1·061	1·386	1·886	2·920	4·303	6·965	9·925	31·598
3	·137	·277	·424	·584	·765	·978	1·250	1·638	2·353	3·182	4·541	5·841	12·924
4	·134	·271	·414	·569	·741	·941	1·190	1·533	2·132	2·776	3·747	4·604	8·610
5	·132	·267	·408	·559	·727	·920	1·156	1·476	2·015	2·571	3·365	4·032	6·869
6	·131	·265	·404	·553	·718	·906	1·134	1·440	1·943	2·447	3·143	3·707	5·959
7	·130	·263	·402	·549	·711	·896	1·119	1·415	1·895	2·365	2·998	3·499	5·408
8	·130	·262	·399	·546	·706	·889	1·108	1·397	1·860	2·306	2·896	3·355	5·041
9	·129	·261	·398	·543	·703	·883	1·100	1·383	1·833	2·262	2·821	3·250	4·781
10	·129	·260	·397	·542	·700	·879	1·093	1·372	1·812	2·228	2·764	3·169	4·587
11	·129	·260	·396	·540	·697	·876	1·088	1·363	1·796	2·201	2·718	3·106	4·437
12	·128	·259	·395	·539	·695	·873	1·083	1·356	1·782	2·179	2·681	3·055	4·318
13	·128	·259	·394	·538	·694	·870	1·079	1·350	1·771	2·160	2·650	3·012	4·221
14	·128	·258	·393	·537	·692	·868	1·076	1·345	1·761	2·145	2·624	2·977	4·140
15	·128	·258	·393	·536	·691	·866	1·074	1·341	1·753	2·131	2·602	2·947	4·073
16	·128	·258	·392	·535	·690	·865	1·071	1·337	1·746	2·120	2·583	2·921	4·015
17	·128	·257	·392	·534	·689	·863	1·069	1·333	1·740	2·110	2·567	2·898	3·965
18	·127	·257	·392	·534	·688	·862	1·067	1·330	1·734	2·101	2·552	2·878	3·922
19	·127	·257	·391	·533	·688	·861	1·066	1·328	1·729	2·093	2·539	2·861	3·883
20	·127	·257	·391	·533	·687	·860	1·064	1·325	1·725	2·086	2·528	2·845	3·850
21	·127	·257	·391	·532	·686	·859	1·063	1·323	1·721	2·080	2·518	2·831	3·819
22	·127	·256	·390	·532	·686	·858	1·061	1·321	1·717	2·074	2·508	2·819	3·792
23	·127	·256	·390	·532	·685	·858	1·060	1·319	1·714	2·069	2·500	2·807	3·767
24	·127	·256	·390	·531	·685	·857	1·059	1·318	1·711	2·064	2·492	2·797	3·745
25	·127	·256	·390	·531	·684	·856	1·058	1·316	1·708	2·060	2·485	2·787	3·725
26	·127	·256	·390	·531	·684	·856	1·058	1·315	1·706	2·056	2·479	2·779	3·707
27	·127	·256	·389	·531	·684	·855	1·057	1·314	1·703	2·052	2·473	2·771	3·690
28	·127	·256	·389	·530	·683	·855	1·056	1·313	1·701	2·048	2·467	2·763	3·674
29	·127	·256	·389	·530	·683	·854	1·055	1·311	1·699	2·045	2·462	2·756	3·659
30	·127	·256	·389	·530	·683	·854	1·055	1·310	1·697	2·042	2·457	2·750	3·646
40	·126	·255	·388	·529	·681	·851	1·050	1·303	1·684	2·021	2·423	2·704	3·551
60	·126	·254	·387	·527	·679	·848	1·046	1·296	1·671	2·000	2·390	2·660	3·460
120	·126	·254	·386	·526	·677	·845	1·041	1·289	1·658	1·980	2·358	2·617	3·373
∞	·126	·253	·385	·524	·674	·842	1·036	1·282	1·645	1·960	2·326	2·576	3·291

SOURCE: This table is taken from Table III in Fisher and Yates: *Statistical Tables for Biological, Agricultural and Medical Research*, Published by Longman Group, Ltd. London (previously published by Oliver & Boyd Ltd. Edinburgh) and by permission of the authors and publishers.
a. n = degrees of freedom.

TABLE A4
Distribution of χ^2

Probability.

n^a	·99	·98	·95	·90	·80	·70	·50	·30	·20	·10	·05	·02	·01	·001
1	·$0^3$157	·$0^2$628	·00393	·0158	·0642	·148	·455	1·074	1·642	2·706	3·841	5·412	6·635	10·827
2	·0201	·0404	·103	·211	·446	·713	1·386	2·408	3·219	4·605	5·991	7·824	9·210	13·815
3	·115	·185	·352	·584	1·005	1·424	2·366	3·665	4·642	6·251	7·815	9·837	11·345	16·266
4	·297	·429	·711	1·064	1·649	2·195	3·357	4·878	5·989	7·779	9·488	11·668	13·277	18·467
5	·554	·752	1·145	1·610	2·343	3·000	4·351	6·064	7·289	9·236	11·070	13·388	15·086	20·515
6	·872	1·134	1·635	2·204	3·070	3·828	5·348	7·231	8·558	10·645	12·592	15·033	16·812	22·457
7	1·239	1·564	2·167	2·833	3·822	4·671	6·346	8·383	9·803	12·017	14·067	16·622	18·475	24·322
8	1·646	2·032	2·733	3·490	4·594	5·527	7·344	9·524	11·030	13·362	15·507	18·168	20·090	26·125
9	2·088	2·532	3·325	4·168	5·380	6·393	8·343	10·656	12·242	14·684	16·919	19·679	21·666	27·877
10	2·558	3·059	3·940	4·865	6·179	7·267	9·342	11·781	13·442	15·987	18·307	21·161	23·209	29·588
11	3·053	3·609	4·575	5·578	6·989	8·148	10·341	12·899	14·631	17·275	19·675	22·618	24·725	31·264
12	3·571	4·178	5·226	6·304	7·807	9·034	11·340	14·011	15·812	18·549	21·026	24·054	26·217	32·909
13	4·107	4·765	5·892	7·042	8·634	9·926	12·340	15·119	16·985	19·812	22·362	25·472	27·688	34·528
14	4·660	5·368	6·571	7·790	9·467	10·821	13·339	16·222	18·151	21·064	23·685	26·873	29·141	36·123
15	5·229	5·985	7·261	8·547	10·307	11·721	14·339	17·322	19·311	22·307	24·996	28·259	30·578	37·697
16	5·812	6·614	7·962	9·312	11·152	12·624	15·338	18·418	20·465	23·542	26·296	29·633	32·000	39·252
17	6·408	7·255	8·672	10·085	12·002	13·531	16·338	19·511	21·615	24·769	27·587	30·995	33·409	40·790
18	7·015	7·906	9·390	10·865	12·857	14·440	17·338	20·601	22·760	25·989	28·869	32·346	34·805	42·312
19	7·633	8·567	10·117	11·651	13·716	15·352	18·338	21·689	23·900	27·204	30·144	33·687	36·191	43·820
20	8·260	9·237	10·851	12·443	14·578	16·266	19·337	22·775	25·038	28·412	31·410	35·020	37·566	45·315
21	8·897	9·915	11·591	13·240	15·445	17·182	20·337	23·858	26·171	29·615	32·671	36·343	38·932	46·797
22	9·542	10·600	12·338	14·041	16·314	18·101	21·337	24·939	27·301	30·813	33·924	37·659	40·289	48·268
23	10·196	11·293	13·091	14·848	17·187	19·021	22·337	26·018	28·429	32·007	35·172	38·968	41·638	49·728
24	10·856	11·992	13·848	15·659	18·062	19·943	23·337	27·096	29·553	33·196	36·415	40·270	42·980	51·179
25	11·524	12·697	14·611	16·473	18·940	20·867	24·337	28·172	30·675	34·382	37·652	41·566	44·314	52·620
26	12·198	13·409	15·379	17·292	19·820	21·792	25·336	29·246	31·795	35·563	38·885	42·856	45·642	54·052
27	12·879	14·125	16·151	18·114	20·703	22·719	26·336	30·319	32·912	36·741	40·113	44·140	46·963	55·476
28	13·565	14·847	16·928	18·939	21·588	23·647	27·336	31·391	34·027	37·916	41·337	45·419	48·278	56·893
29	14·256	15·574	17·708	19·768	22·475	24·577	28·336	32·461	35·139	39·087	42·557	46·693	49·588	58·302
30	14·953	16·306	18·493	20·599	23·364	25·508	29·336	33·530	36·250	40·256	43·773	47·962	50·892	59·703
32	16·362	17·783	20·072	22·271	25·148	27·373	31·336	35·665	38·466	42·585	46·194	50·487	53·486	62·487
34	17·789	19·275	21·664	23·952	26·938	29·242	33·336	37·795	40·676	44·903	48·602	52·995	56·061	65·247
36	19·233	20·783	23·269	25·643	28·735	31·115	35·336	39·922	42·879	47·212	50·999	55·489	58·619	67·985
38	20·691	22·304	24·884	27·343	30·537	32·992	37·335	42·045	45·076	49·513	53·384	57·969	61·162	70·703
40	22·164	23·838	26·509	29·051	32·345	34·872	39·335	44·165	47·269	51·805	55·759	60·436	63·691	73·402
42	23·650	25·383	28·144	30·765	34·157	36·755	41·335	46·282	49·456	54·090	58·124	62·892	66·206	76·084
44	25·148	26·939	29·787	32·487	35·974	38·641	43·335	48·396	51·639	56·369	60·481	65·337	68·710	78·750
46	26·657	28·504	31·439	34·215	37·795	40·529	45·335	50·507	53·818	58·641	62·830	67·771	71·201	81·400
48	28·177	30·080	33·098	35·949	39·621	42·420	47·335	52·616	55·993	60·907	65·171	70·197	73·683	84·037
50	29·707	31·664	34·764	37·689	41·449	44·313	49·335	54·723	58·164	63·167	67·505	72·613	76·154	86·661
52	31·246	33·256	36·437	39·433	43·281	46·209	51·335	56·827	60·332	65·422	69·832	75·021	78·616	89·272
54	32·793	34·856	38·116	41·183	45·117	48·106	53·335	58·930	62·496	67·673	72·153	77·422	81·069	91·872
56	34·350	36·464	39·801	42·937	46·955	50·005	55·335	61·031	64·658	69·919	74·468	79·815	83·513	94·461
58	35·913	38·078	41·492	44·696	48·797	51·906	57·335	63·129	66·816	72·160	76·778	82·201	85·950	97·039
60	37·485	39·699	43·188	46·459	50·641	53·809	59·335	65·227	68·972	74·397	79·082	84·580	88·379	99·607
62	39·063	41·327	44·889	48·226	52·487	55·714	61·335	67·322	71·125	76·630	81·381	86·953	90·802	102·166
64	40·649	42·960	46·595	49·996	54·336	57·620	63·335	69·416	73·276	78·860	83·675	89·320	93·217	104·716
66	42·240	44·599	48·305	51·770	56·188	59·527	65·335	71·508	75·424	81·085	85·965	91·681	95·626	107·258
68	43·838	46·244	50·020	53·548	58·042	61·436	67·335	73·600	77·571	83·308	88·250	94·037	98·028	109·791
70	45·442	47·893	51·739	55·329	59·898	63·346	69·334	75·689	79·715	85·527	90·531	96·388	100·425	112·317

SOURCE: This table is taken from Table IV in Fisher and Yates: *Statistical Tables for Biological, Agricultural and Medical Research*, Published by Longman Group, Ltd. London (previously published by Oliver & Boyd Ltd. Edinburgh) and by permission of the authors and publishers.
NOTE: For odd values of n between 30 and 70 the mean of the tabular values for $n - 1$ and $n + 1$ may be taken. For larger values of n, the expression $2\chi^2 - 2n - 1$ may be used as a normal deviate with unit variance, remembering that the probability for χ^2 corresponds with that of a single tail of the normal curve.
a. n = degrees of freedom.

BIBLIOGRAPHY

Alwin, D. F. (1978). *Survey design and analysis: Current issues*. Beverly Hills, CA: Sage.

Babbie, E. R. (1973). *Survey research methods*. Belmont, CA: Wadsworth.

Bennet, A. E., & Ritchie, K. (1975). *Questions in medicine*. London: Oxford University Press.

Berdi, D. R., & Anderson, J. F. (1974). *Questionnaire design and use*. Metuchen, NJ: Scarecrow.

Blalock, H. M. (1972). *Social statistics* (2nd ed.). New York: McGraw-Hill.

Campbell, D. T., & Stanley, J. C. (1963). *Experimental and quasi-experimental designs for research*. Chicago: Rand McNally.

Day, R. A. (1979). *How to write and publish a scientific paper*. Philadelphia: ISI Press.

Frey, J. H. (1983). *Survey research by telephone*. Beverly Hills, CA: Sage.

Johnson, A. (1972). *Social statistics without tears*. New York: McGraw-Hill.

Johnson, E. D. (1982). *The handbook of good English*. New York: Facts on File.

Kidder, L. H. (1981). *Research methods in social relations* (4th ed.). New York: Holt, Rinehart & Winston.

King, L. S. (1978). *Why not say it clearly? A guide to scientific writing*. Boston: Little, Brown.

Kirk, R. E. (1968). *Experimental design: Procedures for the behavioral sciences*. Belmont, CA: Brooks/Cole.

Kosecoff, J., & Fink, A. (1982). *Evaluation basics*. Beverly Hills, CA: Sage.

Labow, P. (1980). *Advanced questionnaire design*. Cambridge, MA: Abt Associates.

McIver, J. P., & Carmines, E. G. (1981). *Unidimensional scaling*. Beverly Hills, CA: Sage.

Siegel, S. (1956). *Nonparametric statistics for the behavioral sciences*. New York: McGraw-Hill.

Slotnick, H. B. (1982). Interviewing turtles and tortoises in malls. *Evaluation and the Health Professions, 5*, 245-258.

Strunk, W., & White, E. B. (1962). *The elements of style*. New York: Macmillan.

Tuckman, B. W. (1972). *Conducting educational research*. New York: Harcourt Brace Jovanovich.

Tukey, J. W. (1977). *Exploratory data analysis*. Reading, MA: Addison-Wesley.

Ullman, N. R. (1978). *Elementary statistics: An applied approach*. New York: John Wiley.

INDEX

ABOUT THE AUTHORS

Arlene Fink, Ph.D., and **Jacqueline Kosecoff,** Ph.D., have been partners for ten years. They are directors of Fink and Kosecoff, Inc., a company specializing in health services research and policy, program evaluations, and other research methods. They are also Adjunct Associate Professors of Medicine and Public Health at UCLA.

Drs. Fink and Kosecoff have coauthored numerous articles and books. Among their publications are *An Evaluation Primer* (Sage, 1980) and *Evaluation Basics* (Sage, 1982).